CW01082950

Active Australia is abou
become more involved in
and physical activity. The framework, developed in
collaboration with state and national agencies,
provides a common direction in making Australia a
healthier and more active nation.

Mark McKeon's book, *Every Day Counts*,
encourages people to become healthier, more
productive and generally enjoy life more. It
complements the Active Australia message by
promoting enjoyable and achievable levels of
physical activity. Research shows that being active
is a key step toward improving health, well-being
and quality of life. *Every Day Counts* and Active
Australia both demonstrate the benefits of being
physically active well beyond those related to
increased strength, endurance, mobility and weight
control. Social, emotional and economic benefits are
also realised by increased activity.

Active Australia wholeheartedly recommends
Every Day Counts. It is an entertaining, friendly
and easy-to-use approach to building physical
activity into our lives and helps us to monitor our
progress.

EVERY

DAY

COUNTS

SO COUNT EVERY DAY

Mark McKeon

Mark McKeon.

HarperCollins*Publishers*

For Carole, Jake and Sam – the ones who count the most.

HarperCollins*Publishers*
First published in Australia in 1999
Reprinted in 2003
Reprinted in 2008
by HarperCollins*Publishers* Pty Limited
ABN 36 009 913 517
A member of HarperCollins*Publishers* (Australia) Pty Limited Group
www.harpercollins.com.au

Copyright © Mark McKeon 1999

The right of Mark McKeon to be identified as the moral rights
author of this work has been asserted by him in accordance with
the *Copyright Amendment (Moral Rights) Act 2000* (Cth).

HarperCollins*Publishers*
25 Ryde Road, Pymble, Sydney, NSW 2073, Australia
31 View Road, Glenfield, Auckland 10, New Zealand
77–85 Fulham Palace Road, London W6 8JB, United Kingdom
2 Bloor Street East, 20th floor, Toronto, Ontario M4W 1A8, Canada
10 East 53rd Street, New York NY 10022, USA

National Library Cataloguing-in-Publication data:

McKeon, Mark.
    Every day counts! So count every day : your system for a
    healthy body and balanced lifestyle.
    ISBN 0 7322 6520 7.
    1. Exercise. 2. Nutrition. 3. Stress mmanagement.
    4. Lifestyles – Health aspects. I. Title.
613

Also by Mark McKeon:
Work a Little Less, Live a Little More

Mark McKeon's Life Tips
www.markmckeon.com

Set in 10/13 Sabon
Cover photograph: The Image Bank/Philip Porcella
Printed and bound in Australia by Griffin Press on 79 gsm Bulky Paperback

Foreword

The quest for health and fitness is consuming the thoughts and actions of a large majority of people in our society. More education about what can be good for us and, more importantly, what is bad for us has led to a multitude of programs suggesting ways to a satisfactory level of personal health and wellbeing.

Most of these programs aren't clear on exactly how you are supposed to reach your goal. None that I have seen until now have provided a daily system that continually measures, monitors and nurtures your progress. I believe Mark's Every Day Counts system is unique in that it provides a day-by-day method, presented in a manner that can be easily understood by us all.

Having worked with Mark for more than 10 years as a player and coach at the elite level of AFL football, I have the highest regard for his work. I have seen him implement programs that have ensured that players reached their potential in their physical and mental preparations. Of course, these programs would be too arduous for the average person: elite athletes require elite preparations.

Mark has a passion for helping people achieve the level of fitness that is right for them. He constantly spreads the word and lives the example about finding the path to personal health. He finds it hard to understand why people would inflict the damage they do on their own bodies, and I have no doubt that this frustration was a factor that contributed to the writing of this book.

Mark's system is simple, concise and self-driven, without the spartan constraints of some programs. The daily points system is easy to work with, informative and motivational. I'm sure you will also enjoy Mark's humorous anecdotes, which bring to life the principles he is so committed to.

We all want the ability to control our own destinies. This book can give you control of your own personal fitness and wellbeing, and show you how to measure it. I congratulate Mark on his foresight in making his system accessible to everyone who wants to achieve a healthy lifestyle.

Tony Shaw
Senior Coach
Collingwood Football Club

Contents

Preface

'All things are difficult before they are easy.'

JOHN NORLEY

TOMORROW NEVER COMES

Everything you've ever tried to keep yourself balanced, fit and healthy, right up until opening the cover of this book, is in the past. Welcome to your future.

It was the Englishman, Joseph Collier, who summed up one of life's great ironies. Collier started the United Drapery chain from an investment of just 50 pounds and built an international conglomerate. He accumulated wealth, prestige and power throughout a frantic working life only to find that his most prized asset had deserted him. He said shortly before his death, 'In this drive of mine to expand, I'm afraid I've neglected my health. It's the only thing I still want, and I can't have it.'

What a way to define remorse. Too many people spend years waiting for a bolt of lightning to come out of the sky and motivate them to change to a more balanced way of life. They are waiting for a BFO (a blinding flash of the obvious). American TV host Oprah Winfrey experienced her BFO while she was watching a Mike Tyson fight some years ago. When Tyson was introduced at 230 pounds, Oprah suddenly realised that she was exactly the same weight as the heavyweight champion of the world. It was a BFO for her that it was time to make some changes, and to her credit, she has.

We cannot depend on divine intervention. You can spend your life waiting for a BFO that may never come.

By the time Joseph Collier realised his mistake, it was too late. Life isn't a dress rehearsal. This is it.

There are steps you can follow to the body and mind you've always wanted! This is your invitation to the Health Zone — an invitation to live the life you want to live, without feeling that you're always compromising one area of your life to satisfy another. You can manage a company and still manage your weight, raise a family, develop your mind, spend time with your friends and yes, be fit, healthy and balanced all at the same time.

TAME THE TREADMILL

'It's not just the years in your life,
it's the life in your years.'

THE DELUGE OF DELUSION

I often think that the way we live resembles a pendulum. Our moods change, eating habits vary, activity patterns ebb and flow, even our general level of happiness with life is constantly swinging from side to side. We rarely stay in one place for very long!

At one end of life's pendulum swing there is what I call *delusion* and at the other extreme there is *illusion*. In the centre is the Health Zone. That's where we are heading.

At the *delusion* end of the pendulum's swing people deny that there is any connection between lifestyle, morbidity and mortality. They dispute that the way we live makes any difference either to our day-to-day vitality or the overall length of our lives. They'll tell you about an uncle who smoked until he was 88, drank whisky for breakfast and died only when his parachute failed to open. They'll also try to convince you that they are happy 'just the way they are'.

Think of the busiest day you've ever had, then imagine every day being this frantic. For people like this, life is a continual rush. If you don't hurry up and finish what you're saying, they'll interrupt and finish it for you. They're waiting for someone to invent a microwave fireplace so they'll be able to sit in front of the fire all night in five minutes!

You can recognise these people when they are driving. You'll see the mobile phone in one hand, note pad in the other and steering wheel between their knees, as they fly past you on the wrong side of the road. To them a stop sign is just a suggestion, traffic is a competition and traffic lights are an abomination. They are in a serious hurry. They live life the same way they drive.

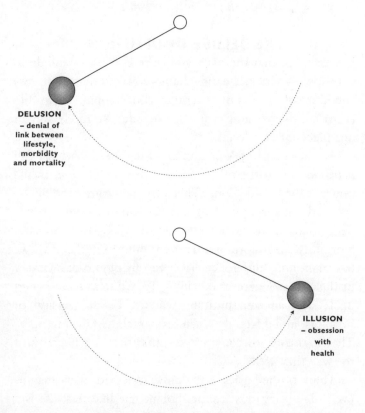

DELUSION
– denial of link between lifestyle, morbidity and mortality

ILLUSION
– obsession with health

Imagine putting yourself under this sort of pressure, pressure that pushes the stress button in the pit of your stomach, wakes you at night and makes you fret about your future. Think of a time in your life when your every waking thought was dominated by anxiety. It's work all week, then sleep all weekend just to try to catch up. Life in the fast lane is a *delusion*. If you think you can handle it, then you're not thinking straight. Even heroin addicts think they can handle their habit. Watch out — that light you see at the end of the tunnel could be the train coming.

We don't set out willingly to combine constant stress with constant body abuse; it just evolves until we're trapped into living each day of our lives this way. People can exist like this, but it seldom lasts for too long. The best advice I can give you if you live at this extreme on the lifestyle pendulum is not to start reading any long books ... you may never get to the conclusion!

If people at the *delusion* end of the pendulum's swing were having a great time, I could understand why they wouldn't want to change! Make no mistake though, we're not talking here about happy and relaxed people with a carefree attitude of living each day as it comes. We're talking about stressed people who have neglected their health. These people often suffer from tight chests, shallow breathing, lack of energy, afternoon fatigue, pallor, lethargy, reliance on artificial relaxants, rashes, twitches, bad breath, poor sleeping habits ... and no charisma!

Your behaviour doesn't even need to be extreme for you to live on the *delusion* side of the lifestyle pendulum. Apathy and inactivity are different types of *delusion* but they are just as lethal. Lots of people are so sedentary that they don't even burn the candle at one end! They fade out rather than burn out, and in one third of cases, their very first indication of heart disease is sudden death! Without overstating the obvious, sudden death tends to take all the fun out of life. Why go through life so worried about your health that you're afraid to buy green bananas because you're not sure you'll still be around by the time they ripen?

Of course, the real attraction of healthy living is vitality. It's not just how long we live that's important, it's how well we live. It's not just the years in your life, it's the life in your years. It's how well we feel, how happy we are and how much we achieve each day of our lives.

People devote their youth and middle age to achieving financial independence. We should also consider our health independence. Why suffer pain and malaise? Why rely on doctors, surgeons and medicines when we don't have to? Shares, properties and bank balances aren't the only assets to build in life. Building our health assets is the best and longest-term tax and capital-gain-free investment we'll ever make.

When he was well into his eighties, George Burns joked about his age during his stage act by saying: 'If I'd known that I was going to live this long I would have taken better care of myself.' In reality, he did take care of himself! Away from the cameras, George was more at home with cycles than cigars, he was very relaxed and he had a great balance in his life.

All in all, the *delusion* end of the lifestyle pendulum is not a great place to be. People delude themselves into thinking that lifestyle is an irrelevance to health. It's a classic case of not letting the facts get in the way of a good excuse.

THE ALLURE OF OBSESSION

At the other limit of the lifestyle pendulum's swing is obsession with health. It's the *illusion* end. This is when people treat their bodies like temples and try to live every day the way dedicated elite athletes do in the lead up to the most important competitions of their lives.

At this end of the spectrum, fat and alcohol are obscenities, while exercise is mandatory and strictly regimented. Stress management techniques are scheduled into daily life, but they are narrow, inflexible and formal. Think of a Tibetan monk training for the Olympic marathon. Now you start to get a mental picture of when the passion for healthy living becomes an obsession. Like all obsessions, what begins as a passion for health can very soon become an *illusion*.

At this end of the lifestyle pendulum's swing, life is something to be endured rather than enjoyed. Each day's abstinence from the harmful pleasures of life is an achievement to be appreciated and respected, but it's rarely a lot of fun. With this level of commitment, the potential dietary harm you might do to yourself by eating an ice cream rather than an orange is far outweighed by the stress the denial itself causes. The cure is worse than the problem.

Being continually vigilant and never allowing any impurity to pass by your lips is a hard rule to live by. Never missing a day's exercise eventually wears you down, physically and emotionally. There is seldom any spontaneity or enjoyment, only grim stoicism to see it through and rack up another day. Sooner or later you burn out. You either drop it, or it drops you. These are the only choices! You can't make a life out of health fanaticism.

It sounds easy to advise people at this *illusion* end of the spectrum to lighten up and relax, but it's just as hard to heed advice if you're in *illusion* as it is if you're in *delusion*.

What are you trying to be: An example of what to be, or a warning of what not to be? The pendulum keeps swinging, and people keep getting left behind.

FACING FACTS

A 30-year, ongoing study of the highest integrity at the Harvard Medical School has found that an appropriate lifestyle can add, on average, at least two years to an individual's expected life span. Two years may not sound like all that much now, but imagine for a moment that you somehow knew when your time was going to be up. The closer that time came, the more and more attractive another two years would become.

While average life expectancy has increased from 43 years at the turn of the century to currently being around 80 years, this doesn't automatically help the cause of people who live extreme lifestyles. Gains in life expectancy have levelled off considerably over the past two decades and in some countries there has actually been a decline in how long people can expect to survive! Being born in the dawn of the 21st century does not guarantee longevity. An extreme lifestyle may limit your lifestyle.

The reality is that the huge number of premature deaths caused by lifestyle abuse is keeping the average down. It seems that for every person who enjoys good health into their eighties and beyond, there is another who checks out before they even have a chance to develop some grey hair. People in *delusion* and *illusion* are keeping the average down.

Living healthy is likely to provide you with a lot more than an extra two years of life. Chances are your life-span gain could effectively be as much as two decades! Next time you are about to complain about the aging process remember that it is definitely the lesser of two evils!

SICK AND TIRED OF BEING SICK AND TIRED

Doug Carr was never an athlete. I met him in the mid-eighties when he was working for a photographic company. I was conducting a Corporate Health Promotion Program at the plant at the time. Doug was a classic case of all work and no play. He clocked up long hours in the office and had no time to exercise. Our paths crossed when his colleagues convinced him to fill in for a lunchtime volleyball competition.

By the time he was into the second set of volleyball, Doug had realised just how out of shape he really was. There was no spark in his spike and the only digging he was doing was trying to make a hole to hide his embarrassment.

Doug decided to get back into shape. He was fed up with feeling lethargic and off colour. The volleyball may not have qualified as an Oprah Winfrey type BFO, but his physical ineptitude certainly got his attention. He asked me if I would map out a program for him to follow at the company gym during lunchtimes. After a few weeks, as Doug was slowly progressing through his gentle routine, I suggested he incorporate a 5-minute jog-walk into his mid-day sessions.

To help him get started, I offered to tag along. We set off around the plant at a very gentle pace. On that first day we jogged 400 metres and walked about the same distance. Doug found the effort physically fatiguing and mentally disturbing. He was in his late thirties at the time, and he'd been very sedentary over the previous 10 years.

We talked about the way he was spending his life and Doug realised that he had been living at the *delusion* end of the lifestyle spectrum. His inability to do things he previously would have breezed through really made him take stock. He desperately wanted to make a change in his life, so he began training more regularly, seeking my advice on everything from diet and heart rate monitoring to the latest in weight-loss and cross-training techniques.

Within another month, Doug was scheduling daily training sessions. He was finding exercise time he previously just couldn't afford, and within 3 months he was running 10 uninterrupted kilometres. He commented that in the office environment he was more productive than ever. His work efficiency was at an all time high. It was looking like an all around success story. Doug had really taken control of his life. He had swung his lifestyle pendulum away from *delusion* and into a zone of admirable lifestyle balance.

That's when the trouble started! The momentum of his new found energy and wellbeing was becoming a force in itself, a force that would keep Doug right on swinging to the other side of the lifestyle pendulum!

In a classic case of more is better, Doug implemented drastic changes to his routine. No longer would he run two or three times each week and cross train on the other days. Now he simply ran every day because he felt he 'didn't get the same burn' with the more moderate sessions. He not only achieved the target weight we had agreed on; he went 4, 6 and then 8 kilos under it! He was running longer and longer distances and having fewer and fewer rest periods. He began to look haggard and drawn, but he managed to complete his first marathon, taking great satisfaction in his achievement. In the space of just under 12 months, Doug Carr went from being unable to run more than 200 metres to being able to run over 42 kilometres!

This success, at least in Doug's mind, spurred him onto an even stricter running program and an absolutely spartan regime of nutritional sacrifice. A man who was previously so willing to take my advice became obstinate and refused to moderate his training. I really felt as if I had created a monster.

The following year Doug achieved the ambition of many athletes by running a sub 3-hour marathon. An admirable turnaround and an incredible change for the better? Not by my standards. What many applauded as a remarkable achievement over a 2-year period, I saw as an uncontrolled swing to the *illusion* end of the lifestyle pendulum.

Doug had now turned 40 and could run a marathon in under three hours, but he suffered constant leg pain and he had a chronic rasping cough and a nagging persistent cold. He wouldn't admit it, but colleagues told me that Doug's work performance was also suffering. He was back to being constantly tired and hungry again. He was underweight, unhappy and unhealthy. His quality of life was no better than it had been when he was at the *delusion* end of the pendulum. The phrase 'out of the frying pan and into the fire' could well have been coined to describe the turmoil in Doug Carr's life. He had swung from one side of the lifestyle pendulum to the other, and once again he was out of control.

Doug's story is an all too common one. Good intentions are not enough and sometimes the nature of our human psyche is such that the thing we most need protection from is ourselves.

THE POINTLESS PINNACLE

In the centre of the pendulum's swing is a magical point of perfect lifestyle balance. We can achieve this knife-edge of perfect harmony through a combination of factors. It's when we eat low fat until supper and then reward ourselves with a small treat while relaxing at night. It's when we exercise moderately and consistently most days of the week. It's also when we take plenty of time out to allow our subconscious mind to relax us by moving control of our thoughts away from our conscious mind.

Like Doug Carr, too many people spend their lives swinging from one side of the life pendulum to the other. They make a commitment to healthy living by embracing exercise, diet and anxiety control. Unfortunately, the best of intentions is not enough and if their commitments are premature or unrealistic, their lifestyle will deteriorate. They then go into denial and swing wildly back toward the other end of the pendulum, the *delusion* end. It's the classic 'this time it will be different' yo-yo scenario. Commitments are made, broken and remade.

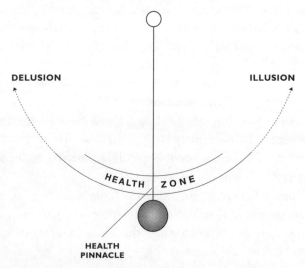

The perfect point of balance is like a Utopian state. It's a narrow mountainous ledge, a great place to try to get to, but a very difficult place to stay for too long. I call it the Health Pinnacle. The problem with the Health Pinnacle is that the pendulum keeps swinging and it's very easy to get knocked off your perch. You can see the Health Pinnacle approaching, you reach it and then before you know it, the momentum pushes you over the edge and back down the slippery slopes to the danger zones of *delusion* or *illusion*.

If you think that I'm going to show you how to live in this absolute mid-point of the lifestyle pendulum, to balance on this knife-edge of healthy living, you're wrong. I have an even better way!

ZEROING IN ON THE ZONE

A decade ago, lack of information was the main reason people let their health prematurely deteriorate. It was ignorance, pure and simple. Over the past 10 years, health agencies across the world have initiated campaigns to educate us about the benefits of exercise, low-fat diets and management of stress. The health message is now all around us. It's everywhere from the sides of cereal boxes to the faces of multi-storey billboards. Everyone seems to know the benefits of relaxation, regular exercise and low-fat eating.

Remember the cartoon character, 'Norm', from the 'Life. Be In It.' campaign. 'Norm', and the healthy lifestyle principles he was associated with, was familiar to 93% of people, but only 12% of people were actually doing anything about it. Even armed with knowledge, which is supposed to be the way to power, only 1 person in 8 was adopting healthy lifestyle practices. Awareness by itself is like trying to row a boat with one oar.

Unfortunately, it's still only a small minority of people who actually manage to put those principles into practice. As a result of those health promotion programs we've increased activity rates of the adult population, though even now it's still only around 18% of adults who exercise regularly and control their diet. It's clear that with less than one in five adults adopting healthy life habits, we have failed to achieve a health-focused community. All the promotional and educational efforts have failed to produce the desired result. The reason is simple.

It's no longer a lack of knowledge that stops us from living the lives we want, it's lack of will to really do it. This book will help you to find that will within you. It will help you get that second oar into the water.

THE TREADMILL OF LIFE

Most of us have the desire to relax and eat well because we know it's good for us, and we squeeze in some time for exercise whenever we can. For many people, it's like being on a treadmill.

Take the case of Louise, a busy office worker who has only 40 minutes for lunch. She races down to the city gym and pumps out exactly 20 minutes on a computerised running machine. The treadmill is equipped with speed and incline controls, a touch screen interface to race whoever's alongside her and Nintendo-like graphics to blast away Super Mario on her own personal screen. The treadmill's electronic buzzer sounds to end Louise's 20-minute workout. There's no time for a cool down so it's a race to the shower, a sandwich gulped down while dressing and a dash to make it back to work on time. She is going from one treadmill to another. It's the treadmill of life.

Living the life you want isn't only about doing the things you think you should do. It's not just what we eat, but how we eat, its not just exercise that's good for us, it's exercise in sync with the rest of our lives. We can never separate the physical and emotional parts of our being. Like it or not, we are a package and we have to live as a package if we are going to tame the treadmill.

You can get more out of yourself: more productivity, more enjoyment, more satisfaction and more vitality. Your life may not be lacking at the moment — in fact I hope your life is great. I just want you to have high goals to make your life the best it can be.

What do I do next?

Think about your goals. I won't be asking you to focus on a point of perfect lifestyle harmony. The Health Pinnacle is very hard to get to and even harder to balance on. That's not the answer.

I want you to live in a state of balance I call the Health Zone. It's the best location in town and it's a great place to spend your time. The system we will use to help you find the Health Zone is called Every Day Counts.

Welcome.

2

HOW THE SYSTEM WORKS

*'Destiny is not a matter of chance,
it is a matter of choice.'*

LEIGH MATTHEWS

SYSTEM COMPONENTS

Every Day Counts is a simple and effective healthy lifestyle system for you to follow each day for 9 months.

There are three components in the Every Day Counts system: food, exercise and pressure. Your task is to achieve a daily points target according to the foods that you eat, the exercise you do and the way you deal with pressure.

Your challenge is develop healthy habits. To do this you are asked to reach your daily targets, first for 7 days, then for 7 weeks and finally for 7 months. The 7 days, 7 weeks and 7 months add up to a total of 9 months. This 9-month system duration signifies a 'rebirth' and will ensure that you develop permanent healthy habits.

You may be used to counting frequent flyer points; now get ready to count health points. It may be useful for you to refer to Appendix 1: Fast track from time to time whilst you're getting the hang of Every Day Counts.

TRANSITION

The most effective way to implement the Every Day Counts system is through a 2-week transition period. Your time starts now! As you read the book I hope you will introduce and experiment with earning food, exercise and pressure points. By the end of the 2 weeks you will have completed the book and experienced enough of the system to be ready to begin in earnest.

IN THE MEANTIME . . .

Here are a few questions I'm regularly asked about the system.

Why should I regiment my life by counting points? It's not as if I don't have enough to do already!

The answer is fundamental and very, very important. If you do not have a system to follow, you won't change! It's as simple as that. My grandmother used to say that the road to hell was paved with good intentions. She was right on the money when it comes to lifestyle habits. Even when you're on the right track, if you're not moving fast enough, you will still get run over.

I've dealt with the health and fitness of elite athletes, children, overweight and overstressed business people and virtually everyone in between. I've worked in the field for almost 20 years. Business people are especially vulnerable because of having a finite amount of time and an infinite number of demands on that time.

Trying to be more efficient with our time is like trying to reduce the amount of paper we use in the office. We may eventually achieve a low pressure, paperless office, though at the moment it's about as likely as a paperless toilet!

There is one striking trait common to all of us: woman or man, girl or boy, we are all creatures of habit. Change is hard to achieve. We revert to our habits because they feel natural to us. The more pressure we're under, the more quickly we look for the comfort these habits bring.

We can change our habits, but we need a system to help us. The system is the bridge that connects intentions and actions. Counting points will help you improve your health habits in the long run, and that's what it's all about.

How long will it take me to work out my points?
It will take you a maximum of 3 minutes each day.

What do I actually have to do?
Your task is to calculate 3 scores each day. These are your food, exercise and pressure scores. You can do this either mentally or in a diary (see Appendix 3). You add the 3 numbers together and that's it, you've scored for the day!

How many points do I have to score each day?
In each week there are 4 exercise days and 3 rest days. You choose when to have your rest days. On exercise days your challenge is to score 12 food points, 4 exercise points and 4 pressure points. Your daily target is therefore a total of 20 points.

On the rest days there are no exercise points. Your daily target is 12 food points and 4 pressure points for a total of 16 points.

You score food points and pressure points every day, while you only score the exercise points on the 4 days each week that you decide to work out.

Do I have to keep doing this forever?
No. The system is designed to become redundant after 9 months. After 9 months you will no longer require the

discipline of Every Day Counts to reinforce your health habits. The positive behaviours will become habitual and you will no longer need the external reinforcement of any system, fitness kick or diet. You won't be on a lifestyle program; it will just be life, life in the Health Zone.

How do I work out my food score?

Every food and drink has a rating of +1 point for a healthy choice, −1 point for an unhealthy choice, or 0 points for a neutral choice. There is a limit to how many food choices you can make in one day. You don't have to go hungry and you won't have to eat bird seed and celery all day. As you progress through the day, you simply keep a written or mental checklist of what you've eaten and the points you've scored accordingly.

FOOD FACTORS

How will I know what foods are good and what are bad? I don't want to carry a book and a calculator around with me everywhere!

You don't have to. You probably have a pretty good idea of good food choice and poor food choice already. By the time you finish the book, you'll be classifying food without even being conscious of it. You'll find all the foods and drinks you are likely to have listed in Appendix 2. Within a week or so of Every Day Counts, you'll need to refer to the food listings only when you try exotic or unusual foods.

Does this mean that I can't eat anything that I like any more?

No. It's important to have some fun in your diet and no foods are totally excluded. Your focus is avoiding excessive fat intake. Fat is the big enemy. We are all at risk from bad food 24 hours a day. For this reason most foods with a high fat content rate a negative score, and if you have too many negative scores, it becomes very difficult to accumulate the points you are aiming at for that day.

Can I make unlimited food choices?

The standard number of daily food choices is 25. An apple counts as 1 choice, a cup of coffee counts as 1 choice, a dinner of meat and 3 vegetables counts as 4 choices. Anything up to 200 grams is 1 choice. A large steak, for example, weighing 300 grams, would count as 2 choices.

You may opt to have more or less food and drink choices (30 choices if you weigh more than 90 kilograms or 20 choices if you weigh less than 55 kilograms). The rule of thumb is you need a net score at the end of the day of half the number of total choices you make. People making 30 food choices need to reach a food score of 15. Thirty food choices are the absolute maximum. No one needs more than 30 food choices a day.

People making 20 food choices each day need a net food score of 10 points. While most people find that 25 food or drink choices a day is the right level, you can adjust the number to suit your needs.

Please do not starve yourself. Making 25 food choices a day does not mean you will put on weight. As long as you achieve your food points target as well as your exercise and pressure points target, you will not put on fat!

Can you give me a couple of examples of 'positive' and 'negative' food choices?

Ice cream and chocolate rate as −1 point because they are high-fat, poor choices, while apples, high-fibre bread, brown rice and other good foods rate as +1 point. Some foods, like mineral water and tofu, are neutral and rate as 0. Your daily food target is 12 points.

You are able to score 2 extra food points by further limiting your negative food choices. You can use these points if you have a deficiency in your exercise or pressure score for that day. Fourteen points are your maximum food score on any day.

Even if you somehow managed to score 18, 20 or 25 food points, your maximum claim for food for that day is restricted to 14 points. In other words, you can't score extra by taking the system to extremes or eliminating fat completely. Our system embraces three components of lifestyle balance. Healthy eating by itself is not enough. In fact, no single behaviour can dominate. If we allowed that, we'd be encouraging lifestyle *illusion* and we'd be right back where we started.

You can get away with a couple of poor choices each day. You will still achieve 12 daily food points even when you have a couple of negative scores. In fact I will be encouraging you to make bad food choices because living in the Health Zone allows you to enjoy food for taste as well as for health.

Wouldn't it be easier to just try and cut out bad food choices? Then I wouldn't have to count points all the time!

Tennis star John McEnroe always said he found it harder to close the fridge than to close out a tough five-setter. If athletes find it almost impossible to maintain food discipline when they rely on willpower alone, what hope do we have? We need to follow a system to control our food intake; otherwise it will control us. It's a case of eat, drink and be wary!

Do I buy packaged low-calorie food as part of the program?

Definitely not! You don't need to rely on packaged, home-delivered food that tastes like cardboard, and we don't have to force ourselves to pay hundreds of dollars to a weight loss clinic just so we feel committed to stick with their program. If weight control is an issue in your life, Every Day Counts will help you.

Don't feel that you always have to eat the right thing. Some breakfast cereals, especially a few of the high-fibre varieties, do nothing else but make you wish it was already lunchtime. You know the ones: they don't go snap, crackle or pop, they just suck up all the milk and sit there! That's no fun. When you reach your daily food points target by Every Day Counts, you'll be getting all the fibre you need.

How do I decide whether something is 1 or 2 food choices? Is bread with butter 1 choice or 2? What about a big steak? Is that still 1 choice even though it's much bigger than a slice of bread?

Good question. You do need to consider the size of your choices. Anything up to 200 grams in weight is considered to be 1 choice; 200 grams is approximately the same size as the palm of your hand. A large steak of 350 or 400 grams will count as 2 choices. A slice of bread is wider than the palm of your hand but it is thin and weighs less than 100 grams; it's 1 choice. If you have butter on the slice of bread, the combined weight is still under 200 grams so the bread and the butter together still count as 1 choice.

When you have something good, something +1 (like bread) with something –1 (like butter) together in one food choice, because it's still under 200 grams, do I count it as a +1 for the bread, a –1 for the butter, or do they cancel each other and make a 0?

A plus and a minus together cancel each other out and make a 0. Remember that the system requires you to get

12 points from your 25 choices. If you have too many 0 or –1 choices, you'll struggle to build up the required points.

What about big and small eaters? Surely not everyone should eat the same quantity?

Twenty-five food choices are your recommended level. Large-framed people who weigh in excess of 90 kilograms may need up to 30 food choices per day. Small-framed people who weigh less than 55 kilograms may need as few as 20 food choices per day.

Don't, however, confuse appetite with hunger. Appetite applies to what we get used to eating. Without food our stomach is no larger than the size of an orange. To accommodate a large meal, desserts, drinks and 'afters', it can swell to the size of a basketball. If we are in the habit of overeating and keeping our stomach full, when the stomach starts to empty and shrink it sends appetite pains to the brain. You genuinely feel hungry, but what you are really feeling is appetite, not hunger. Hunger pains tell us what we really need.

How can you tell the difference? Take all your clothes off and stand in front of a mirror. Jump up and down five times, then stop suddenly and start counting. If there is anything still wobbling by the time you've counted to three, you will know that you've being responding to appetite rather than to hunger!

Seriously, if you are a 'big eater' weighing between 55 and 90 kilograms, you need to find out if you have a big appetite or a big hunger. Try 25 food choices for a week or so. You may be surprised to find that you don't need as much as you thought you did. Your aim is not to go hungry and a large intake of good quality food seldom causes weight problems. It's fat that fools.

Drink a glass or two of water before you eat. This will partially fill your stomach and reduce the need for food filling. Eat slowly. Part of our psychological make-up tells us that the longer we've been eating the more we must have eaten. A good chew of each mouthful helps digestion and allows you to gain the full nutritional value of the food.

Slowly reverse your overeating trend by having smaller serves, especially for dessert. Your stomach will adjust and you will avoid the situation where your appetite causes you to eat a lot more than you need.

Can you give me an example of a day's healthy eating that will score the 12 points I need?

Breakfast: cereal (1), low-fat milk (1), fruit (1), wholemeal toast with jam (1), juice (1), water x 500 ml (1)

Morning tea: banana (1), juice (1)

Progress score = 8 points

Lunch: 2 x salad sandwiches on rye, no butter (2), muffin (–1)

Afternoon tea: orange (1), 500 ml water (1)

Progress score = 11 points

Dinner: large wholemeal pasta (2), neapolitana sauce (0), 2 × vegetables (2), yellow cheese (–1), tofu (0), water (1), coffee with sugar (1) and two sweet biscuits (–1)

Daily food score = 15 points

Food and drink choices = 23

In this example, you could make 2 more food choices, both negative, and still achieve your target for the day. The system allows you the chance to eat treats like chocolate or ice cream or to indulge your taste buds. If God wanted us to eat only steamed white rice, we wouldn't have taste buds. Every Day Counts simply keeps you in control and in balance.

WORKING OUT YOUR WORKOUTS

Why do I have to count points for exercise? Can't I just work out without having to remember my score?

Exercise is the closest thing we will ever have to a universal panacea. Even so, exercise for most people is what they are going to do next year.

I've been involved with an elite Australian Football Club for almost 15 years. A few years ago we started what we called the 'gym option' where members of the club could pay a fee and have access to the same facilities and training advice as the players. The overwhelming response from the corporate members was that they would be happy to pay $200 each to be involved, but they'd be even happier to pay $300 to say they were involved, just as long as they didn't actually have to come along! That's what it's like with exercise. It sounds like a good idea, but when it comes right down to it, it's not that comfortable, you get all sweaty, people look at you as if you are demented and it takes up so much time.

We need more than an exercise principle. We need a system that will overcome inertia and a lifetime of on-again-off-again exercise habits. This time you'll actually be able to do it.

So how do I score exercise points?

Counting exercise points is very straightforward. Points are awarded on the basis of training time rather than training intensity or speed. You score 1 point for each 15 minutes of exercise you do. Fifteen minutes is the minimum period that will you earn a point!

All exercise rates the same. Walking scores the same as running, tennis, squash, swimming, gardening, kite flying, stretching and circuit training. It's all 1 point per 15 minutes. Six points, which equate to 90 minutes of training, are your daily exercise maximum. You can use these 'extra' points if you earn them, to make up for a shortfall in your food or pressure points on that day.

How many exercise points do I need each day?

You need 4 points, which is the equivalent of 1 hour on the exercise days, and no points on any of the 3 rest days.

If I do an extra hour of training, could I have 4 more negative food items? Please tell me I can do extra training to make up for a bad food day!

It is possible to score only 8 food points and try to make up the shortfall with 2 extra exercise points (on exercise days) and 2 extra pressure points. This is designed to give you some leeway to stay in the Health Zone. However, on the non-exercise days when you can't score exercise points, you will have to be more disciplined with your food and pressure points to reach your overall target.

How do the rest days work?

I don't want you to exercise every day. Your body needs rest as well as training to benefit from your efforts. On 3 days each week your total target score is 16 points rather than 20 points. Remember that you cannot score any exercise points on these days. While you are free to train on these days if you wish, you cannot earn any exercise points to contribute to that day's target.

Can you give me an example of a day's exercise that would enable me to score the 4 points I need?

A daily exercise routine of a 45-minute morning walk (3 points) followed by a 15-minute stretch (1 point), would give you the 4 points you need. A 60-minute bike ride would achieve the same result.

PRESSURE POINTS

Why do I have to score pressure points?

Controlling anxiety is the link between our physical being and our emotional being. You will be developing an important skill, a skill that will enable you to choose your own thoughts. Pressure is okay; you can even make it a positive. It's stress that's the negative. Pressure becomes stress only when we allow it. We'll show you how to stop pressure becoming stress. That's why you are counting pressure points rather than stress points. Prevention is better than cure.

Even though it may sound straightforward, the principle of stress management is both the easiest and the hardest of our three health factors. Let me show you what I mean. Please consider the jumble of letters below:

sbixanleatntearss

Can you delete 6 letters from this list and leave an easily recognisable English word? Now delete 10 letters and leave exactly the same English word? It seems an impossible task to delete both 6 letters and 10 letters and still leave the same word. It can be done, if you choose your thoughts!

How could this be so? The answer is at the foot of the page so please spend a couple of minutes trying to solve the dilemma before reading on.

Here's the answer. The only possible way you can delete 6 letters and 10 letters at the same time is to delete the words 'six letters'. It takes 10 letters to write 'six letters' so the answer looks like this:

b a n a n a s

Congratulations if you solved the puzzle.

What's the point?

Lateral thinking problems like this rely on our subconscious mind to exert some influence over our conscious thoughts. Day by day, we very rarely give our subconscious mind a chance to contribute to our lives. We are so focused on climbing the corporate ladder, keeping the house as neat as we can, or making the first-grade team, that we never give our goals and ambitions a rest. We put a lot of pressure on ourselves. It's the 'dumb and dumber' approach to life. I can imagine you nodding your head as you read this. It's true and we all do it!

It's the subconscious mind that helps us relax, reduces our blood pressure, slows and deepens our breathing rate and decreases muscle tension. The subconscious mind helps us to switch on by switching off. It allows us to change our focus from operational to strategic and to use our minds to get the best out of our bodies.

Ever solved a problem or remembered an answer when you weren't really trying, perhaps when you were thinking about something else? That's your subconscious mind breaking through the barriers put up by your conscious mind. My secondary school English teacher always advised our class to invest five minutes of exam time in daydreaming. Her theory involved reading the essay or exam topic and then deliberately ignoring it for the next five minutes. This simple strategy makes a lot of sense. Even though the exam time pressure was severe and every minute was crucial, taking this five minutes was an effective use of time. We were allowing the thoughts to come rather than trying to force them. It worked for our class — but then again we'd been practising daydreaming for years!

Taking time out is the hard part. Once again, this is exactly why we need a system and not just an intention.

So how do I score pressure points?

You score 1 point for every 5 minutes spent keeping your life in balance. It means taking time out, nothing more, nothing less. You can use relaxation techniques like progressive muscular contractions and relaxation, deep breathing, tai chi, prayer, meditation, sensory deprivation, massage, spa or sauna. Anything that helps you to switch off will promote physical and mental harmony. Think of it as food for the soul.

Your target is 4 pressure points each day, so you will have to invest 20 minutes of your precious time. You have the ability to score up to 6 points each day by allocating an extra 10 minutes to controlling pressure. This gives you some flexibility to make up for a deficiency in your food or exercise points if you happen to come up short on any given day.

Of course you are welcome to spend more than 30 minutes enjoying the benefits of this vital area if you wish, though you can't score or 'claim' more than 6 points. A 20-minute mental imagery session or the same time spent in a spa is enough to achieve your target for the day. It's a 4-point pressure refresher!

Before you know it you really will be choosing your own thoughts!

Can I make up a deficiency in one area by earning exra points in one of the other two?

You can't make up for a major deficiency in one area by over-emphasising the other two, but you do have some leeway. A marginal eating day might score only 10 points, but you could make up the difference by attaining extra exercise or pressure points. We are looking for a Health Zone rather than an absolute Health Pinnacle.

Food points:	Target = 12	Daily maximum = 14
Exercise points:	Target = 4	Daily maximum = 6
Pressure points:	Target = 4	Daily maximum = 6

So what's my overall daily target again?

Twelve food points, 4 exercise points and 4 pressure points will give you your daily target of 20 points on the exercise days. On the 3 non-exercise days your target is 12 food points and 4 pressure points for a total of 16 points.

What is the maximum I could score in one day?

You can actually score up to 14 food points, 6 exercise points and 6 pressure points on a daily basis. It's therefore possible to score up to 26 points overall on a day when you have exercised. This 'perfect score' of 26 points (or 20 points on a non-exercise day) is *not* your goal. Please remember that you are striving for the Health Zone, you are *not* aiming for the Health Pinnacle.

Why is nutrition worth more than exercise and stress control?

While all three areas are vital, food is the area we have to work on hour by hour. It takes one decision to do an exercise workout and it takes one or at the most two decisions to take some pressure time during the day. When it comes to food, however, we have to make as many as 18 correct decisions every day. We need around 18 × '+1' food choices to make up for the inevitable –1 food choices we will make along the way. We need hourly vigilance to succeed in the battle against food and that's why it's worth so many points.

What will the system do for me?

The system will provide you with a daily reminder of how to live a balanced lifestyle and achieve peak performance in life, sport, business and in any other area you have a passion for. If you take too many short cuts, you'll fall short of your points target for that day. You cannot ignore any of the three vital areas.

HUMANITY DAYS

What do I do if I don't make my target for a day?

Try again the next day. I encourage you to use a 7/7/7 rewards system to help you overcome the obstacles you will face. This means you receive a reward every day for the first 7 days after commencing the program. You then receive a reward every week for the next 7 weeks and finally every month for the next 7 months.

Your rewards must all be planned in advance. To begin, plan to treat yourself to 7 daily rewards when you reach your daily points targets. Buy a magazine, hire a video, call a friend long-distance, do anything that will give you a boost. It may only be a token but a little positive reinforcement goes a long way.

To make the task even more realistic, you only have to achieve your daily points target on 6 out of 7 days each week. The 'day off' is what I call your humanity day. Effectively, it's one day each week when you are allowed to fall short of your target. Please do not treat this as a complete binge day. It's not an excuse to turn your back on your principles and over-indulge. Think of it as a realistic acceptance that sometimes things won't go as planned. It's an additional incentive to keep with the program.

Humanity days do not fall on the last day of each week; they are there to use when you need them. It could be the first day of one week, the third day of the next week and the sixth day of another week. In many weeks you won't need a humanity day at all, and in case you are wondering, *No*, you definitely cannot hold them over or save them up. Don't use it just because it's there. Use your humanity day when you need it.

Once you're through the first 7 days and have enjoyed your first 7 rewards, you then receive a reward at the end of each week for the next 7 weeks. Going out to dinner works well, while some people prefer to buy CDs, books or other material self-rewards.

After 7 successful weeks, your rewards become monthly. Now you have to invest in yourself. Buy yourself some clothes, a new gadget or a weekend away. Use your imagination and reward yourself with things that really mean something to you. The reward system is one more way to motivate yourself to stick with the program through the inevitable highs and lows. Remember — plan all 21 rewards (7 daily, 7 weekly and 7 monthly) before you start your first day on the Every Day Counts system.

The humanity days mean that you only have to reach your daily points target on 6 out of 7 days as you progress through each calendar month. When you reach your daily target on 6 days out of 7, you have earned your reward for that week. Take it. Remember, don't use your humanity day as an excuse to go ballistic; it's a way of fostering your goals of self-control, moderation and enjoying the good things in life.

The reward system is a once only offer and if you have a setback you have to work your way back to where you were to earn your next reward. If you happen to fall short of your target on the sixth day, and you have already used up your humanity day on the third day, you will have to start again at the beginning. You must succeed for another 6 days before you can claim your sixth daily reward.

Any time you fall short of your target more than once in a week, you are back to the very beginning. It's tough and fair and the only way to make the system truly effective in changing your habits. At all times you have to get back to where you were to achieve your next incentive. The system gives you enough leeway to keep your humanity and show some human frailty, yet still succeed. It effectively allows you to lose your balance without falling off the wagon. If you feel shaky, use your humanity days as a type of wheel alignment to get you back on track. Don't let the wheels fall off completely.

The longer you stay with the system, the more motivation you'll have to keep on staying with it. That's why the rewards start daily and then progress to weekly and eventually monthly. If you can make it through the first month, the hardest part will be behind you.

The 7 days, 7 weeks and 7 months collectively add up to 9 months. When you follow the system for 9 months, you'll no longer need it at all. It's almost like a rebirth. If you are a parent, you will know the ultimate and indescribable joy of a new life you have created. Here's a chance to create a new life for you.

While on the subject of kids, I once worked with a young dad called Rob. Rob had poor health habits along with the worst health habit of all, smoking. (By the way, I won't specifically mention smoking in this book, but if anyone contacts me with questions, I'll answer the questions from smokers first, because smokers have much less time left than the rest of us!) Rob's family was very keen to see him make some changes and they offered to assist in any way they could. With his family's help, we devised a 7/7/7 rewards system to provide the incentives Rob needed. This is how it worked.

For the first 7 days, Rob's wife agreed to make mad passionate love to him every night if he kept to the system and reached his targets. When he first heard of the suggestion, Rob quipped that it would be no different to any other week, but he very quickly decided he'd take up the offer!

His 7 weekly incentives were also mapped out in advance. They included nights out at the movies and dinner, car washes, some toiletries, a book, and a dad's day when the kids had to obey Rob's every wish for three hours.

The monthly rewards were also planned. Rob and his wife had a weekend getaway; he bought himself new car seat covers, a fishing rod and some work boots, and the family got involved with a theme park visit and a new computer game. The money spent on rewards came through the savings from less take-away food and no cigarettes.

The rewards have to mean something to you, and you must commit to taking them when they are achieved. There is nothing more self-destructive in the long run than earning a reward and then not taking it.

Rob made it. He now eats well, trains moderately and he has conquered his nicotine addiction. His family loves his new found vitality and Rob is quick to tell the tale of how his life is so much better for the changes he has made. Even so Rob keeps looking for something else to change so he can go through that first week again!

What do I do next?
The next few chapters will give you all the information you'll need about food, fitness and fighting stress. If you're desperate to begin now, you'll find comprehensive food tables and an Every Day Counts diary in Appendixes 2 and 3, though I hope you'll stick with us and not jump too far ahead. There's a lot more to talk about.

Let's get started.

3

MAKING THE UNHEALTHY EATING CHOICE

'People with no vices have very few virtues.'

ABRAHAM LINCOLN

THE UNHEALTHY CHOICE

I recently witnessed first hand the hilarious irony in how some people make their food choices. I was conducting Teambuilding and Communication sessions at the National Funeral Directors Annual Convention. The funeral directors told me that it is wise to stay fit and lively in their industry, otherwise you run the risk of getting mixed up with the stock.

As part of the program, the National Heart Foundation held a morning walk and healthy breakfast session, complete with an educational address from the eminent cardiologist, Dr Don McTaggart. There were also two senior representatives of the National Heart Foundation present.

You may think that the Heart Foundation and the Funeral Directors Association are on opposite sides of a life and death issue like heart disease. One is trying to keep people alive while the other is always on the look-out for new business! However, the Funeral Directors Association is a great supporter of the Heart Foundation. It is now very common for people to request donations be made to the Heart Foundation instead of sending flowers to funeral services. This provides an important source of funds for the Foundation's ongoing work. Besides, the average person falls ill and recovers fifteen times during a lifetime. It's the sixteenth time that causes the problem.

Back to the convention. Only 15 people out of the 180 convention delegates took part in the morning walk. While this was a disappointing turnout, it was even more disappointing that amongst the absentees were both executives representing the Heart Foundation itself. They didn't make it to their own early morning walk! Admittedly it was the morning after a St Patrick's Day function and a few Guinesses had been downed at the previous night's convention dinner. Fortunately, although they missed the walk, the Heart Foundation executives did make it to hear Dr McTaggart speak and to enjoy what was supposed to be a healthy breakfast. Numerous other convention delegates had also arrived for a feed by this time even though they had slept through the walk.

It was ironic to watch many of the walkers, most of the non-walkers and even one of the Heart Foundation executives ignoring the fruit, cereal and pancakes on offer, and instead attacking heaped plates of bacon, fried eggs, sausages and hash browns. If this was their idea of a 'healthy heart' breakfast, I'd hate to see what they had other mornings.

This feeding frenzy was going on at exactly the same time that one of the country's leading cardiologists was speaking about risk factors associated with heart disease, and emphasising the role of healthy nutrition. At one point Dr McTaggart moved around the tables holding up a small model of the heart and its blood vessels to demonstrate just how fine the coronary arteries really are and what happens when they become blocked. As he moved closer so people could inspect his model, one of the bacon demolishers was so engrossed in his plateful of food that for a moment he thought he was being offered a salt shaker. Luckily he realised his mistake in time and withdrew from the movement of reaching up to accept what he thought was more salt. He was already adding fat to his arteries. Had he accepted the model he would have been adding arteries to his fat! It was farcical. Here we had a cardiologist, a man who spends every day trying to repair the damage caused by food abuse, in the very act of pleading for lower fat nutrition, while most of the people present, including one of the National Heart Foundation leaders, couldn't stop themselves, not even for one day, from gorging on fat.

SUICIDE BY DRIP FEED

The same sort of people as those at the convention will in years to come bemoan the way their health has deserted them. They will look back in failing health and wonder, 'What did I ever do to deserve this?'

Heart disease is no accident. It happens because most people poison themselves with fat for 40 years. Slowly but inevitably their blood vessels become clogged. Someone is having a heart attack somewhere in Australia every 10 minutes. (As the joke goes, that 'someone' must be getting sick of it by now.)

The experience at the Funeral Directors Convention convinced me once and for all that information alone does not help people make the right food choices. Information without commitment is useless. People try to contribute toward a healthy diet because they want to do the right thing; they just lack the real commitment to actually do it. It's as motivators say: 'I'm not interested in your commitments, I'm interested in your commitment to your commitments.'

What will it take to really get you committed, really commmmitted? You already know how to differentiate between fatty food and low-fat food. Unfortunately, there is nothing more ineffectual than good intentions and bad food. It's like committing suicide by drip feed. Every Day Counts is the bridge between contributing and committing. (Do you know why the difference between bacon and eggs is like the difference between contributing and committing? Well, the hens are contributing, but the pigs are committed!)

I imagine that underfed people in developing countries would be happy to get their hands on whatever food they can, and who would blame them? For many unfortunate people, food isn't about health; it's about survival. For the rest of us, despite what some people may say in bluff or jest, there isn't a person on the planet who wouldn't like to eat well if they could somehow find a way of doing it instead of just wishing it.

Bad food choices are the result of either ignorance or an inability to resist what we are conditioned to eat. We just can't get past the temptation of our taste buds. Poor eating is created out of habit and habits are hard to change. The people at the Heart Foundation's healthy breakfast are just one more example. The Funeral Association Convention delegates are far from being unique. Very few people are single-minded enough to eat the right foods all of the time. We alternate between being strong and giving in when the craving for fatty food becomes irresistible, then eating poorly and feeling guilty. It's all too easy to dig our graves with our knife and fork. Every Day Counts provides the link between good intentions and good eating.

FROM CONTRIBUTING TO COMMITTING

Believe it or not, making some unhealthy eating choices is exactly what you should be doing. We can neither deny nor eliminate our urge to eat fatty food, though we can control it. Making one or two unhealthy eating choices daily will satisfy your urge to eat foods that tempt with taste then fool with fat. These choices will count as negative choices and move your score in the wrong direction. However, you will more than make up for these over the course of the day by making the majority of your food choices positive ones.

Occasional poor choices will not create weight or health problems. They will allow you to keep control. Sometimes bad can be good.

The Every Day Counts system also provides a psychological advantage. You don't feel guilty when you treat yourself to a chocolate bar or a croissant for no reason other than it tastes good. You've seen people hiding biscuits in the backs of their hands or walking into the office with their faces so full of corn chips that they can't open their mouths to answer a question. Psychologically, they are rationalising that if no one else notices the bad food, they won't either. It's much better to occasionally indulge than to compulsively obsess.

Easy to say, hard to do, right? It's hard because trying to understand nutrition has become complicated as trying to wade through the superannuation laws. The so-called authorities have clouded food and health research with confusing jargon and contradictory concepts. Food values are prone to different interpretations. Like our superannuation laws, which seem to change annually, as soon as we hear that a particular food is good or bad for us, a new recommendation is announced and it's often completely the opposite of the previous dogma.

There is a solution: think about grams when you think about fat!

DON'T GUESS ON GRAMS

Every time we eat we are faced with choices. At breakfast we can choose fat-filled butter or fat-free jam to put on our toast. For a morning snack we can choose chubby cheese or a fat-free apple. When we order pasta from a restaurant menu, it's our decision whether to select a fatty cream-based sauce or a fat-free tomato-based sauce. We almost always have a choice.

The Golden Rule is to make the right choice, most of the time. The way to do this is to count grams. Do not count calories or kilojoules, do not count protein or carbohydrate, and forget about things like food density and glycaemic index. Just think *grams* when it comes to fat. When you are unsure about whether a food choice is going to be a +1 or −1, ask yourself: 'How many grams of fat are there in this food?' Read the label to find out how many grams of fat you'll be taking in or check the listings in Appendix 2.

As long as your total fat intake for the day is between 40 and 50 grams, you won't tally up too many negative food points and you'll still be getting the amount of fat that you do need. Less than 40 grams of fat is too little; more than 50 grams is too much. It's a narrow range, but when you keep your fat content between 40 and 50 grams each day, you'll know that you are on target! Think of a darts board. The further you stray either way from the 40 to 50 grams range, the more you'll move away from the bullseye to the outer rims of your target.

When you eat between 40 and 50 grams of fat and you score the 12 food points required within our Every Day Counts guidelines, you will be protecting your health and boosting your vitality.

You'll enjoy the extra energy you'll find living in the Health Zone. Once you experience this feeling it will be all the motivation you'll need to reinforce the 40–50 grams of fat per day habit. You won't let this feeling go.

All foods can be classified as carbohydrate, protein or fat. When your fat intake is under control, you don't need to concern yourself with monitoring carbohydrates and protein. As long as you're not starving yourself altogether, the all important factor is keeping your fat content between 40 and 50 grams per day. If you're taking in only a small quantity of fat, carbohydrate and protein must be making up the rest of your diet. There is nothing else the food could be. When you understand this, you're already a long way toward simplifying what you should and shouldn't be eating.

The alternative is to measure carbohydrate, protein and fat every day. This is tough and not something I advise unless you are a dedicated athlete. We often prescribe in athletes' programs that they should consume up to 10 grams of carbohydrate per kilogram of body weight per day. For an athlete weighing 80 kilograms, this corresponds to an amount of 800 grams (80 kg × 10g = 800g) of carbohydrate each day. Protein intake for the same athlete should be around 1.5 grams per kilogram of body weight per day (80 kg × 1.5g = 120g). Fat intake should only be 0.5 grams per kilogram of body weight per day (80 kg × 0.5 g = 40 g).

Measuring and weighing all your food for protein, carbohydrate and fat content can be a nightmare and takes a truckload of self-discipline. It's almost impossible to eat out, you can't plan your final meal of the day until you've totalled up what you've eaten until that point, and you tend to have a lot of unavoidable food wastage. It's very tough socially, financially and logistically. Eating becomes a metabolic chore rather than a source of nourishment and enjoyment. Can you imagine trying to fit this into a family routine, a business schedule or a social life? Don't do it. Why measure all 3 when we only have to monitor 1? Monitor your fat by counting grams and the rest will take care of itself: 40–50 grams per day is the rule to eat by.

Please don't think that you will need a comprehensive knowledge of the fat content in food to do this. You won't. When people are first introduced to Every Day Counts, they are often worried that they will have to carry a book around with them to know which foods score what points. You won't need this. The tables in Appendix 2 give every food a plus, minus or zero rating and they show you how many grams of fat each food contains per 100-gram serving. The tables will give you a guide to refer to when required, though in reality most of us tend to eat the same things over and over. Unless you are an exception to the rule, you prefer to have similar breakfasts and lunches on most days. Most people tend to have more variation in their evening meals, but overall it's fair to say that 'we repeat what we eat'. You also have your favourite drinks and favourite snack foods, and it's also more than likely that there are some foods that you can't stand the taste of and so never eat them. Take Parmesan cheese — I mean take it as far away as you can. I know a lot of people like that stuff, but please, I couldn't get past the smell to eat it even if I wanted to. We all have our likes and dislikes and this narrows things down.

It won't take long before you have a clear understanding of positive, neutral and negative food choices. Chances are you could score most eating choices right now, even without looking at the tables.

Monitoring fat is the key, and Every Day Counts is the simplest and most effective way to achieve this. With Every Day Counts, you are guaranteed to be eating the right amounts of fat, protein and carbohydrate. It's a sure thing.

You may have heard about artificial fats like polydextrose and cellulose. These are sometimes used in frozen treats to lower the fat content while still trying to present a taste like fat. There is also a new product called 'Olestra' which is a combination of sugars and fatty acids. Olestra tastes like fat but can't be digested so it passes through your system virtually gram free. Sounds okay, doesn't it? The problem is it makes everything else pass through your system, too, and in a big hurry! Don't stray too far from a comfort station for the next few hours! There are all sorts of side-effects associated with fat substitutes and we have no idea of what the long-term effects will be. Forget the magic tricks; short cuts are of no more value in your diet than shortbreads!

SU-MUCH FOOD

This is another alternative approach to controlling your diet, but it's not one that I would recommend. It's the Sumo wrestler approach. In the Sumo system, food intake is monitored by the physical weight of the raw food eaten by these massive athletes each day. The Sumos deliberately eat high volumes of fat in order to maximise their bulk. They are issued with 5-kilogram parcels of food to get through each day. That's 5 kilograms, 5000 grams of food every day!

If the Sumos were sticking to our plan of no more than 50 grams of fat per day, that would leave 4950 grams from carbohydrate and protein. This is impossible. The Sumos are obviously taking in a lot more fat, perhaps as much as a kilogram of fat every day. Sumos seldom live much beyond 40 years of age. Every Day Counts is a better option!

Food really does make that much difference, and that's why it earns you 12 points.

FOODS, FATS AND FOLLY

I often have the pleasure of conducting healthy lifestyle workshops for corporate groups based on the Every Day Counts program. During these sessions, I ask the participants the following question: 'What do you think the percentages of fat are in skim, "low fat" and full cream milks?' The consensus from most of the participants who are still awake is that skim milk is 1% fat, low fat milk like Rev or Shape is 2% fat and whole milk is 4% fat. The majority is fairly certain of the last figure because they have seen a television advertisement promoting whole milk. The advertisement displays a vertical scale not unlike a thermometer. As the camera pans downward along the scale, milk is highlighted as being only 4% fat and therefore a low-fat eating choice along with fruit, bread and rice.

The participants at the seminars are initially satisfied when I confirm the facts. Skim milk actually has no fat, zero, and zero means zero. Low fat milk has between 1% and 2% and whole milk has 4%. These figures seem to confirm these beliefs and the numbers sound relatively low. Unfortunately the real facts are hidden!

Brands like Trim, Physical and Rev are between 1% and 2% fat. This is where the confusion starts. These percentages refer to the weight of the milk, not the kilojoules or the grams they contain. If you put 1 litre of 1% fat milk on weighing scales, it's true that only 1% of the weight would be fat. Unfortunately, 1% of the weight does not mean 1% of the kilojoules or 1% of the grams! One per cent of the weight really means 12% of the fat or 10 grams of fat. Milk with 2% fat by weight is really 24% fat by kilojoules and 20 grams of fat. Whole milk, which is around 4% fat by weight, is actually 48% fat by kilojoules and 40 grams of fat.

A food that has 4% of fat does not mean it is only 4 grams of fat.

At this point I've usually woken my seminar audience, but they are well and truly confused, so don't worry if you feel exactly the same way right now. The thing that really counts is grams of fat. When you think grams, you can forget about all the rest.

Let's delve back into the milk mystery. Here's a table showing the grams of fat content per litre of milk, along with kilojoules (kJ) and weight comparisons.

Milk type	Fat per litre	% Fat by weight	% of kJ
Skim milk	0 g	0	0
1% fat milk	10 g	1	12
2% fat milk	20 g	2	24
4% milk (whole milk)	40 g	4	48

When I explain these figures, the seminar-goers challenge me. They have seen the television commercial comparing the fat content of whole milk, at 4%, to fruit, vegetables and rice. How can 4% suddenly become so much more? Unfortunately you can't believe everything you see on television. The technical point about milk being 4% fat is correct because the milk promotion people are measuring by weight. They are morally wrong because the only thing that counts is grams. A litre of milk weighs 1 kilogram. One kilogram is equal to 1000 grams. Four per cent of 1000 grams is 40 grams. That's how 4% by weight can be a whole lot more than 4% when it comes to the true fat.

At my last seminar there was a stunned silence from the audience at this point. I was about to press on when someone asked, 'If the fat is 40 grams, what do the other 960 grams consist of to make up the kilogram of weight?'

I answered that while carbohydrates and protein make up a small amount, the majority of the weight is in the liquid itself, water if you like. It's the same with all foods. Much of the weight comes from the water content. Even the human body is more than half water by weight.

'What about calories, kilocalories and kilojoules?' someone will usually ask.

The answer is that calories and kilocalories are the same thing. Kilojoules are the metric equivalent. There are 4.5 kilojoules in one calorie. Kilojoules are not measured in the same manner that weight is measured. There are 40 kilojoules in 1 gram of fat. There are only 20 kilojoules in 1 gram of carbohydrate and 20 kilojoules in 1 gram of protein. There is a difference because fat is much denser than carbohydrate or protein. (We have to be pretty dense to eat too much fat.)

'So how do you sort through all the confusion?'

Don't focus on fat percentages. They just confuse the issue. Don't think about carbohydrates or protein because they are only half as dense as fat. That's why they only have half as many kilojoules per gram. Protein and carbohydrate will look after themselves.

Fat is the absolute key to controlling your diet rather than letting it control you. Fat has twice the density of protein or carbohydrates and that's why it has so many kilojoules. It's loaded. Forty grams of fat may not sound that much; however, in the example of milk, it's equal to almost half the total kilojoules contained in that litre of fluid. It's also almost equal to a full day's recommended allowance of fat.

The way to control your fat intake is to count your fat intake. This means counting fat grams.

We've been tracking a small group of people who have been using Every Day Counts for more than a year. They have lost an average of 4 kilograms of body weight, 6 points of systolic blood pressure and 4 beats in their resting heart rates. While nutrition is only one third of the Every Day Counts formula, counting food points on a day-to-day basis is a great start to finding your way into the Health Zone.

When 1 litre of milk is enough to provide close to a full daily allowance, you can imagine how much fat some people eat over a full day. Here are a few more examples.

Food	Grams of fat
100 g chocolate	27
fruit museli bar	5
small packet of corn chips	up to 15
quarter skinless barbecued chicken	15
chicken drumstick	10
slice of bread	up to 1
slice of garlic bread	up to 6
butter	16 per tablespoon
hot thin sliced chips	around 32 per 100 g
100 g peas or beans	less than 1
average slice chocolate cake	18
50 g nuts (depending on type)	20–25
slice pizza	15

meat pie or sausage roll	24
200 g rump steak	around 36
trimmed of fat and grilled	less than 20
boiled egg	6
avocado	40–50

Water contains no grams of fat. It carries nutrients, removes wastes, controls body temperature and helps keeps our joints lubricated.

Fat content will vary according to the specific quality of the food you are eating. The key to remember is that it doesn't take long for grams of fat to add up. Your fat consumption target when Every Day Counts is 40–50 grams of fat.

I have counselled hundreds of people who had fat intakes in excess of 250 grams per day. The record (Sumo wrestlers excepted) was an average of 440 grams per day. Notice the past tense? Most people are well and truly above 100 grams every day of their lives. There are lots of Australians with higher averages than Sir Donald Bradman, and that's the reason very few of them get anywhere near a century.

ANOTHER REASON TO SACK FAT

Do I have you convinced yet? I want to leave you with no option in your mind other than to monitor and maintain your fat intake levels between 40 and 50 grams per day. Here's another reason. All food uses a part of the energy it contains to convert itself into a useable form of energy. You may be aware that some nutrients are lost when food is cooked. It's the same thing when we again 'cook' the food we eat to use as energy.

In the case of carbohydrate, 25% of its own energy is used as the carbohydrate is metabolised into what is known as glycogen, a 'ready-to-use' energy form. We effectively have only 75% of the energy to burn off because 25% is used up just getting it ready.

Fat is already in a storable format. If you like, it has been 'pre-cooked' for energy usage. It takes only 4% of the available energy to store fat. That means 96% of the energy contained in fat has to be burned off. It's a double whammy! If you are about to attack half a dozen donuts, remember that fat also has twice as much energy as carbohydrates to start with. Carbohydrates have 4.5 calories per gram, fat has 9 calories per gram.

No wonder they say, 'A minute on the lips, a year on the hips!'

REALITY BITES

Helen is a successful corporate manager. We met at a time when she was having trouble maintaining her desired weight. Her frustration was at boiling point because even though she was far from being a big eater, her weight was creeping up by a couple of kilograms each year. At 168 centimetres, 67 kilograms and 36 years of age, she was concerned about her health, her self-esteem and her corporate image.

I asked Helen to keep a basic food diary for a couple of days. Initially she resisted the idea because she felt she couldn't eat any less than she currently was eating. She had convinced herself that her problem was a combination of a metabolism that was slowing down a little each year, fluid retention and some sort of undeserved curse.

Eventually Helen agreed to keep a diary for just one day. This is her record of food intake for that day. I have added columns on the right for the fat content in grams and for Helen's Every Day Counts food points.

Food intake	Fat (g)	Points
6.30 a.m.		
half glass pineapple juice*	0	+1
1 slice of toast with butter**	5	0
1 breakfast bar	6	0
coffee*, milk and sweetener	3	+1
10.00 a.m.		
black coffee*, milk and sweetener	3	+1
2 × small dry biscuits	6	−1
1.30 p.m.		
1 cup Thai chicken curry	22	−1
1 small slice of garlic bread	7	−1
handful peanuts	8	−1
café latte*, 1 sugar	4	−1
5.00 p.m.		
1 glass Riesling*	0	+1
1 water cracker with cheese	8	−1
8.00 p.m.		
microwave pasta with carbonara sauce		
and sliced avocado (small serve)	25	−1
3 slices of canned peaches	0	+1
black coffee*, milk and sweetener	3	−1
11.00 p.m.		
1 cup of soy milk	9	0

*The first two cups of tea, coffee, fruit juice or alcoholic drinks each day count as +1 points. Additional choices count as −1 point each time.
**A + and a − together, for example bread with butter, cancel each out to create a 0.

Total food choices over the course of the day = 16
   (maximum choices allowed = 25)

Total fat intake = 109 grams (recommended intake 40–50 grams)

Every Day Counts food points = −3 points
   (recommended points target = 12 points)

Helen's total fat intake for the day was 109 grams. Even though her total kilojoule intake was low and she had made only 16 food choices, the proportion of those kilojoules coming from fat was too high. Helen had the full range of misconceptions about calories, kilojoules, fat by weight and fat percentages.

All Helen needed was to be shown these figures on paper, then offered some alternatives that wouldn't turn her life upside down. Helen experimented with counting grams and scoring points every day. Below is a random day taken from her diary, four weeks after she started Every Day Counts. It's interesting to compare this to her original day's food diary.

Food intake	Fat (g)	Points
half glass pineapple juice	0	+1
1 slice of toast with jam	1	+1
1 breakfast bar	6	0
coffee, skim milk	1	+1
10 a.m.		
apple	0	+1
1 glass water	0	+1
1 small dry biscuit	3	−1
1.30 p.m.		
sate beef × 2	8	0
1 warm bread roll	1	+1
diced carrot snack	0	+1
café latte, skim milk	2	+1
1 glass water	0	+1
5.00 p.m.		
1 glass Riesling	0	+1
1 water cracker with cheese	8	−1
1 glass water	0	+1

8.00 p.m.

microwave pasta with Napoletana sauce	4	+1
ice cream × 2 scoops	10	−1
1 glass water	0	+1
half peach	0	+1
200g low fat yoghurt	2	+1

11.00 p.m.

1 cup skim milk	0	+1

These were Helen's 'new' results:

    Total food choices for the day = 21 (previously 16 choices)

    Total fat intake = 46 grams (previously 109 grams)

    Every Day Counts food points = 13 points (previously −3 points)

I knew that Helen was on her way into the Health Zone. She needed a goal to focus on and a system to help her get there. 'As soon as I started counting grams and scoring each food choice with a plus, minus or zero, things started taking care of themselves,' Helen said. 'I was actually able to eat more food while I was losing weight. Every time I make the right choice I think of it as a reality bite.'

Helen now works on 40–50 grams of fat each day and is back in her ideal weight range. She has also found that because she is able to eat more, she has more energy and is therefore more inclined to exercise after work.

'I was in the rut of the century,' she said, "I felt I was eating less and less, and I just kept putting on weight. I just couldn't find the energy to do a workout. I was so miserable. Now I've lost 6 kilograms, going on 7, and I'm walking or swimming every other day. As long as I keep my total points over 20 (food + exercise + stress), I know I've had a good day.'

Helen has some great attributes; she is intelligent, confident and ambitious, street wise, very determined and experienced. If someone like Helen was having trouble finding the Health Zone with all her skills, what hope do the rest of us have? Without a system, we're swimming against the tide. With a system you can believe in, like Helen, you too will soon be back in business.

Helen still makes Every Day Count!

A FINAL FAT FACT

The main theme of this chapter has been reducing fat in your life. I'd like to conclude with one more fat fact to think about.

You know the old style block of butter, shaped in a rectangle and about the same size as a human fist? While it used to be known as half a pound of butter, we now think of it as a 250-gram block. This is about the same amount of fat many of us ask our bodies to cope with every day. It's too much. Our bodies just can't cope with it!

Butter is 82 grams of fat per 100 grams, so in a 250-gram block of butter there is over 200 grams of fat. This means that if you are eating 200 grams of fat or more a day, you are eating the equivalent of a block of butter each day of your life. I'm sure you wouldn't sit down and tuck into a butter block as a matter of choice, though effectively that is what you are doing if your fat intake is at this level. Half of the world's population is overweight and 20% are officially obese, according to the World Health Organisation.

When you make Every Day Count, earn your 12 food points, and follow my recommendation of between 40 and 50 grams of fat per day, you'll be guaranteeing yourself a healthier future. So remember that pastries, chocolate, fried and other fatty foods are like a looking at a cheap suit or a rusty car. *They look good from far, but they're far from good!*

What do I do next?

In the next chapter you will discover that there are myths surrounding certain foods that have carried bad reputations for years.

Remember, food facts are more useful than food fads.

Fallacies associated with body shape and body image are often given the status of fact. Remember the *illusion* end of the lifestyle pendulum and learn to recognise limits to your desire for body enhancement.

4

FACTS AND FADS

'Many receive advice, only the wise profit by it.'

FOODS WITH BAD REPUTATIONS

You know what it's like with reputations — they're much harder to get rid of than they are to get. Golfer Greg Norman lost two major championships 10 years ago because of freak shots from his opponents. Ever since he's battled the reputation of being a 'choker' under pressure. Greg is no more susceptible to pressure than any other elite sportsperson. He's since won two majors and he has dominated the number one rating in the world for almost a decade. Still he battles this undeserved label.

It's the same uphill battle when foods are branded with bad reputations. Some foods deserve their taboo status. Others are unfairly criticised as being fat when in reality they are lean. I'd like to see if we can do for these foods what 10 years of fantastic golf has been unable to do for Greg Norman.

POTATOES

Let's start with potatoes. Potatoes are not fattening, that is if we don't spoil them! Potatoes are high in carbohydrate and they don't contain any fat at all. However, anything cooked in fat will contain fat. Here's how poor cooking choices can ruin what started out as one of the best foods there is.

Cooking choice	Fat (g)
100 g boiled potato	0
100 g potato chips (sliced potato cooked in fat)	14
100 g potato crisps (thin sliced potato cooked in fat)	32

In our Every Day Counts rating system, boiled, mashed (watch the butter) or dry baked potatoes rate as +1 point options. When you fry potatoes in fat as chips or bake them in fat for a roast they become a negative food option.

AVOCADOS

Avocados are high in fat but cholesterol free. This might sound confusing, however, not all fat contains cholesterol. Cholesterol comes from saturated fat which, with the exception of tropical oils like palm oil, coconut oil and cocoa, comes from animal sources. Beef fat and butter fat are the classics. Saturated fat is solid at room temperature and only melts when you heat it up.

There are two types of cholesterol and both are found in saturated fat. HDL (High Density Lipoproteins) is the good cholesterol and LDL (Low Density Lipoproteins) is the bad stuff. Apart from the food we eat, we all produce our own cholesterol. It's a white waxy substance that's necessary as a building block for every cell in our bodies. It also aids in vitamin D and sex hormone production, and it can actually help absorb fat.

It's the HDL that can absorb fats and that's why it's good. It's the LDL that clogs the arteries. Next time you have a cholesterol test, ask for a breakdown between HDL and LDL. An overall cholesterol reading of 5 is considered marginal. However, if the majority of that 5 is made up of HDL it's a fantastic result because the good cholesterol is protecting your arteries and keeping them clear. Conversely, if the greater proportion of the 5 is composed of LDL cholesterol, it's an indication that the arteries have already narrowed. (You don't have to give more blood to have this breakdown analysed; it's just an additional test in the pathology lab. So ask for a breakdown. It could save you having one!)

Unsaturated fat comes from nuts, vegetables and seeds. Unsaturated fat is usually liquid at room temperature but fats like margarine are solid because they have extra hydrogen added during manufacture. Most fish oils are also unsaturated fat and therefore better health options than saturated fat. Avocado is a plant food and contains no saturated fat or cholesterol.

There is also monounsaturated fat, which comes from olive, canola and peanut oils. These are the ones to cook with because they may even reduce cholesterol. These are the best health options when it comes to fat. Avocados are high in monounsaturated fat. A large avocado may contain up to 50 grams of fat, which is a full day's total allowance within our system. Because the type of fat found in avocados is unsaturated it does not cause our cholesterol level to rise, but it's still fat. While avocados won't increase your cholesterol regardless of how many of them you have, eating avocados regularly will certainly tend to increase your weight.

Let's assume that your weight is well managed, but high cholesterol is a problem for you. You are conscious of the need to keep some fat in your diet, but you want the fat to be cholesterol free. For you, avocados are a fantastic food choice. Regardless of your cholesterol level, if weight management is a big issue in your life, avocados should be no more than a very occasional treat. To be conservative with this issue, we rate avocados as −1 in our Every Day Counts system.

NUTS

Nuts have a similar story to avocados. They are high in vitamins, minerals, fibre and fat. As in the case of avocados, it's unsaturated, cholesterol-free fat, but it's still fat.

A small packet of peanuts or cashew nuts contains around 50 grams of fat, Brazil nuts aren't far behind and macadamia nuts are even worse. Like avocados, there are only negligible amounts of carbohydrate in nuts, so unless you are looking for a source of cholesterol-free fat, nuts are far from being an ideal eating option.

They have one other disadvantage. Nuts are often eaten as snacks. If you are taking in your total daily allowance of 50 grams of fat in one small snack, it's going to be very tough to stay within our guidelines for the rest of the day. For these reasons, nuts are very much an unhealthy eating choice. While you might fit them into your diet somewhere, they definitely rate as −1 point options in our Every Day Counts system. Try to save some room for fat in your main meals.

CHEESE

Cheese is an entire area in itself, and one that can be confusing, so the key thing to focus on is fat content. Yellow cheese can exceed 40% fat by grams. This means a 100-gram block of cheese could leave you with 40 grams of fat temporarily sitting in your stomach and looking for a more permanent home. Because the fat found in cheese can be high in cholesterol, that permanent home for the fat will not only be on your hips and your behind, but also inside your blood vessels.

The cheese story is not all bad news. Cheese is an excellent source of protein and calcium and white cheeses like ricotta and cottage are excellent options with low-fat contents. Calcium is a big issue. If you don't get enough in your diet, your body will draw it from your bones, eventually leaving them brittle. It's another reason why low-fat white cheeses are absolute +1 choices.

Be cautious about 'low fat' yellow cheeses. Low fat often means *lower* fat. If you start out life as a 40% fat cheese like cheddar (10 grams of fat in 25 grams of cheese) and you reduce your fat content by a third, you still end up with 7 grams fat in 25 grams of cheese. This is still almost 25% fat. Anything over 20% fat is well and truly a high-fat food, so 'lower fat' or 'reduced fat' can still mean high fat! Don't let them fool you with these percentages or low-fat labels. Stick with grams every time. If the label only has a percentage, work out the grams of fat by multiplying that percentage against the size of your serve. If you have 50 grams of cheese and it's 30% fat, you will be choosing $30/100 \times 50 = 15$ grams of fat. If you're not a maths genius or you can't find your calculator, stick with the rule, 'If in doubt, leave it out!'

There are such differences between cheeses that sometimes you'd be better off eating the chalk! We've classified cheeses individually in Every Day Counts, so please choose carefully when it comes to your cheese platter.

BREAD

Bread is the carbohydrate king. It's very similar to potatoes in that by itself it is one of the best food choices you can make. The big problem is what you have with the bread.

Most breads have less than one gram of fat per slice. Another positive is that the same slice of bread will have between 10 and 20 grams of carbohydrate. The beauty of bread is that it's so high in carbohydrate and so low in fat that you get a double bonus with one food choice.

Many foods are good in one way, bad in another. They may be high in protein but also high in fat, or high in calcium but low in carbohydrate. Bread is the true double adapter, high in carbo and low in fat. It's close to being perfect. There is no need to compromise when it comes to bread. Bread with nothing on it is the most undereaten food in Western society.

It's true that whole-grain bread is higher in fibre and other nutrients, but white breads still contain respectable amounts. Bread is not fattening. It is an excellent food option. Our ratings in Appendix 2 include the one or two bread exceptions you need to be wary of.

BANANAS

If bread is the carbohydrate king, bananas aren't far from the throne. Bananas contain no fat. They are high in carbohydrate (15 to 20 grams), potassium and fibre. Fibre isn't something you digest or use as energy itself, it just helps us digest and use the other things we're eating.

About the only bad thing you can say about bananas is that they can give you bad breath for about half an hour after eating them. Despite the social problems this might cause you, they are still very much a +1 point option in Every Day Counts.

Most foods from plants that grow naturally in the ground and are not over-processed after harvest are excellent food options. To eat well, forget the dogma and concentrate on the facts.

TOO LITTLE IS TOO MUCH

Losing too much weight and too much fat can be negative for your health, your performance and your appearance. There is no shortage of sad stories, even tragedies, when it comes to overtraining and undereating. Arguably, the worst of all are the ones that could and should have been avoided.

In the world of fitness and training, we battle daily to control the use of illegal and immoral drugs like steroids and human growth hormones, but our biggest challenge is that we are yet to find a solution to the growing problem of eating disorders. Being underfat is worse than being overfat!

Being healthy, attractive and athletic is a fantastic thing to aspire to and I encourage you to use exercise points and food points to develop the best body you can achieve. This is a great ethic to have in your life. It's the Health Zone.

Some people find it hard to maintain a balanced perspective regarding their own body shape and personal body image. It's the *illusion* end of the lifestyle pendulum. I have met and admired some of the most aesthetic male and female physiques in the world. I can promise you that even some of these elite athletes are dissatisfied with aspects of their bodies. They would prefer to be taller, shorter, heavier, leaner, or to have a different shape. It's part of our nature to undervalue our own assets. The desire for body enhancement should be a positive and motivational force. However, there is a limit to how far you should go. Here are 10 commandments to help keep your body-shaping and eating habits under control. This is how you know where to draw the line and how to realise when you are already over it.

Commandment 1 Never take performance enhancing or body contouring drugs.

Commandment 2 Never make yourself vomit after eating.

Commandment 3 Never try to control the timing of your menstrual cycle.

Commandment 4 Never accept that the cessation of your periods is a normal reaction to training or eating.

Commandment 5 Never allow yourself to be under 10% body fat (male endurance athletes excluded).

Commandment 6 Never ignore three independent people telling you that you have lost too much weight.

Commandment 7 Never lose more than 2% of your body weight in a week.

Commandment 8 Never lock yourself in a room so that no one will see what you're eating. Show the world.

Commandment 9 Never smoke cigarettes.

Commandment 10 Never believe that you can't change the behaviours that in your heart you know are destructive.

Eating disorders can be very complex and it's hard to listen to other people when what you are doing feels so right. Other people's concern can be just another burden for you to carry, but if you read over these commandments a few times, you might find something in there for you.

THE SPOT REDUCTION MYTH

Most of us know somebody who performs hundreds of sit ups each day, trying to trim unwanted kilos from their stomach. Unfortunately, the idea of exercising a particular area of your body so that you can automatically lose weight from that region is a fallacy. Spot reduction, the removal of fatty deposits exclusively from one particular area, just does not happen.

If it were possible, spot reduction would be the ideal way to lose weight. You could choose the areas you wanted to reduce and just exercise those areas. The idea works on the theory that the exercising muscle draws its energy from the nearest source. This theory belongs in the 'the world is flat' category. The nearest source of fat in the abdominal area surrounds the muscle itself. It's the classic spare tyre and you can't lose it by doing sit ups. It would be a lot easier if things worked this way, but in the real world our bodies use up fat stores throughout the body at an even rate, not just from one location.

The spot reduction theory has been examined in great detail. One landmark study designed exercises to be performed using only one arm. The researchers found that the fat loss from the non-exercised arm was exactly the same as that from the exercising arm, proving once and for all that spot reduction did not occur. Numerous other studies have confirmed these findings.

Spot reduction sounds great in theory. The problem is that it doesn't work!

SMOKING

Ninety-seven per cent of people who develop lung cancer are smokers. If your great-uncle Arthur smoked and lived until he was 80, it was just dumb luck. He played Russian roulette with a loaded gun and made it through. Take just 5 minutes to walk through a lung cancer ward and see how many young smokers aren't going to make it to be the subject of Uncle Arthur stories. You should never smoke again.

Smoking hardens arteries, increases blood pressure, reduces lung capacity, affects the liver, costs a ridiculous amount of money and gives you bad breath.

Imagine God coming to you in your dreams and saying, 'If you don't stop smoking, I'm going to take the life of the person you love most in this world!' What would you do? You'd stop. Don't whine about how hard it is to quit, you would find a way. If your child or your spouse were going to die because you smoked, you would find a way. You would stop.

Now imagine God coming to the dreams of the person who loves you the most. In the dream God says, 'If you can't stop your loved one from smoking, I'm going to take her or him away from you.' You would quit to avoid the pain of losing the person you love the most, why wouldn't you quit to avoid the pain of your loved one losing the person they love the most? You.

If a Martian ever lands on Earth, I'd love to see someone try to explain smoking. 'Why do people smoke?' asks the Martian. 'Doesn't it cause dry throat, shortness of breath, yellow fingers and teeth, bad breath, and doesn't it cost a packet for each packet?'

'Yes,' answers the human. 'However, people find it relaxing and it stops them from putting on weight!'

The Martian does some homework and finds out that smoking has been shown to increase nervous tension rather than decreasing it. It also discovers that the initial weight gain that 'quitters' experience is temporary. Some retired smokers put on approximately 2 kilograms in the first 2 weeks. However, after 6 months of smoking cessation there is no significant weight difference between most people's smoking days and post-smoking days.

The Martian disregards these lame attempts to justify the stupidest thing it has ever seen and continues: 'But doesn't it directly cause heart disease and cancers, the two biggest killers in your society?'

'Well ... yes.'

'And hasn't even passive smoking being linked with death?'

'Well ... yes.'

'Then why do people smoke?' asks the intelligent life from Mars trying to find out if there is any intelligent life on Earth.

At last the human answers with some authority. 'Because they are addicted to nicotine. When people crave a cigarette within 30 minutes of waking, it is a physical addiction. When they crave a smoke most when drinking or around other smokers, it is a psychological addiction. A psychological addiction is easier to break than a physical addiction, but either way it can be done.'

At least then the Martian would understand what it was observing, and if you are a smoker, you should understand what you are dealing with. You have an addiction.

Get some help and get a life. Get a life that's yours to keep. A life like Uncle Arthur's is yours only if the bullet keeps spinning around to the right chamber.

As the rich, famous, good-looking, sexy, powerful and very dead Yul Brynner said before his demise from lung cancer, 'Whatever you do in life, don't smoke.'

SUPPLEMENTS: THE A TEAM

The A team in question here is the combination of Antioxidant vitamins and Amino acids. Their value will become clear as you read on.

Our food chain has been corrupted. Chickens are housed under 24-hour-a-day lighting and fed antibiotics and steroids to make them grow bigger and faster. When we eat chicken we're effectively eating those same antibiotics and steroids. This is why we develop resistance and even immunity to the antibiotics that fight infection. It's no wonder we now need double doses of antibiotics to fight germs, if they work at all! (I'm waiting for the day a suspected sports drug cheat introduces the 'chicken defence...' 'No, Your Honour, I haven't been taking drugs, but I have been eating chicken three times a week!')

Fruits are injected with dye and polished with wax so that they have a desirable colour and texture. The very soils we grow our crops in have become degraded. It's no longer possible for these soils to pass nutrients into the plant foods when the nutrients are no longer in the soil itself.

Even organically grown food can be tampered with after harvest. The fruit and vegetables you're eating today may not have seen an orchard for 6 months or more. They've been held in cool storage. Preservatives and additives are everywhere. Genetically engineered food will only make the situation worse.

Post-mortem decomposition will be delayed because we have so much accumulated preservative in us! Rigor mortis will set in but we will still look as fresh as a daisy, at least on the outside. If it keeps going like this, we won't have to worry about ironing our shirts, we'll just put them on and they'll automatically go starched and stiff from all the 'juice' we carry around from the food we eat!

Enough of the bad news. We need help. It's no longer possible to eat a fully nutritious and protective diet without some external help. That help comes from making the right food supplement choices.

Don't rely on nutritional supplements as a cure-all or a substitute for the right eating habits. Supplements are additives, extras that will provide benefits when they are combined with the right eating habits. The advertising will tell you that if you take 2 magic pills morning and night, even without making efforts to eat well, train or protect your body, you'll still end up looking like an Adonis and performing like an Olympian within 14 days ... News flash! It won't happen. There is no magic! Even illegal and unethical aids like anabolic steroids and human growth hormone will work only when they are combined with regular training and the right foods.

The evidence supporting the benefits of using most supplements is almost exclusively anecdotal. Celebrities and athletes offer testimonials about how the supplement has been of benefit to them. While these sound great, benefits have certainly not been proven in reliable scientific trials over time. Most of the people who endorse these products are being paid for their support. I'm not just talking about the more abstract substances like jojoba and royal jelly; I'm talking about herbal extracts, plant roots, seaweed, tree bark, creatine and carnitine, ming gold, inosine, bicarb soda and anything else you can think of.

ANTIOXIDANT VITAMINS
The only supplements that can make claims that stand up to scientific scrutiny are vitamins and amino acids. The Harvard College and University of Pennsylvania are running an ongoing, 3-decade lifestyle study on more than 50 000 of their former graduates. This is the definitive health study of this century. It is professionally organised, it has a very large population sample, it has been running since the early 1960s and there are no commercial interests influencing the outcomes. This is the real thing.

Part of the study has focused on the antioxidant vitamins, A, C and E. Antioxidant vitamins fight the build up of 'free radical' cells, which are essentially highly charged and very active oxygen particles. These free radicals are produced not only through our own daily metabolism; we also ingest them through the food we eat and the polluted air we breathe. Free radicals attack our immune system and are thought to be precursor cells to cancer cells. They also attack our cardiovascular system. The antioxidants fight and destroy these free radicals. In the Harvard study, after 10 years of moderate dosages of antioxidants, there are much lower incidences of heart disease and cancers amongst the group taking the supplements.

In my opinion the researchers have proven that a regular intake of these vitamins does reduce the incidence of heart disease and cancers. These are our biggest killers and the ones against which we need help to protect ourselves.

Vitamin E is especially valuable when we are limiting our intake of fat. About the only potential negative of eating a low fat diet is that you can end up not getting enough vitamin E. The vitamin E included in antioxidants is one way to be sure you are getting enough.

While there have been no reported side-effects as part of the antioxidant study, there is one factor to be aware of: there is an unproven but possible link between very high doses of vitamin A and birth defects. My advice is that for any women considering starting or expanding their family, their dosage of vitamin A should not exceed 500 international units (IU) each day. Otherwise, the recommended intake of the antioxidants is 1000 IU of vitamin E and 1000 milligrams of vitamin C each day. While these can be taken all at once, it is more effective to split the intake into half dosages morning and night.

Vitamin supplements have often been attacked as being an expensive way to merely get some colour in your urine.

The colour is due to surplus and unused nutrients being eliminated via the bladder. I look at it this way. In a best-case scenario the dollar or so a day that I'm spending on antioxidants is protect me against heart disease and cancer. I'm also topping up my daily nutrient intake because I can't always control the quality of the food I'm eating. In a worse-case scenario, I'm spending a dollar a day on 'living insurance'. Most of us take out life insurance so why not have some living insurance. I'm quite happy not to make a claim on either policy! Coloured urine is fine by me.

AMINO ACIDS

Amino acids are the second supplement to consider, especially if you are a sportsperson, if you lead a hectic life, if you sleep less than 6 hours a night or if you are susceptible to chronic fatigue.

Amino acids are the building blocks that, when joined, make proteins. There are 20 amino acids in all. The amino acids fit together in a variety of ways to form what are in effect different types of protein. The amino acids are like bricks that fit together to make many different patterns. Taking the amino acid supplement ensures that you have all of these patterns available when you need them.

Amino acids are classified as being either 'non-essential,' which means that they can be produced by the body, or 'essential,' which means that they cannot be produced by the body or stored. They must be present in the diet on a daily basis.

Three of the 20 amino acids make up what is known as branched chain amino acids. They are isoleucine (Ile), leucine (Leu) and valine (Val). These amino acids are included in many of the commercially available supplements. Once they are swallowed, the body breaks them down into creatine, which is a prime energy source for our muscles during exercise.

A traditional argument against amino acids is that we take in these proteins through the food we eat anyway and therefore supplementation is unnecessary. While it's true that we may have taken in all our requirement of total protein through food, the specific branch chains or combinations of protein that we need may not be available. This is where the specific amino supplements come in, to fill in the gaps in what our daily food has provided for us. In this way, if there are any amino acids missing as a result of inadequate dietary intake, the supplementary amino acids are available to ensure the supply of optimal nutrients.

So what do all these available proteins do for you? They provide energy and strength, and facilitate recovery, and they do not increase weight! However, while energy, power and recovery are the three areas that amino acids can improve through regular supplementation, they will not enhance your strength unless they are accompanied by a thorough and systematic strength training regimen.

The energy and power advantages provided by amino acids derive from the breakdown of the actual protein itself. This is called catabolism. The protein is converted into a substance known as creatine. This is muscle energy in its purest form. There is a similar sounding substance called carnitine, which theoretically can elevate the amount of fatty acids being broken down into energy. The role of basic carnitine, known as L-carnitine, is marginal and unproven while the new type of carnitine, D-carnitine, has a number of unwanted side-effects, such as loss of muscle myoglobin. Don't go anywhere near it.

The recovery factor is achieved by reducing the amount of lactic acid build-up in the muscle. The process is assisted by protein release by the muscle that is in direct proportion to the amount needed. This self-regulation mechanism works by the muscles feeding back to themselves exactly what they need. It's like a car having a spare petrol tank: the reserve tank can be used to fill up the main tank whenever it's needed. Of course this reserve tank will eventually also run out, but if you are taking amino acids every day you'll keep both 'tanks' topped up. You will have a lot more energy and suffer a lot less fatigue.

For sportspeople, it is important that recovery-based aminos be taken before or during exercise so that they have a chance to take effect. Recovery amino acids taken after you work out will not be as effective as those already in the bloodstream when the exercise is actually being done.

Antioxidant products in the Blackmores, Nutriway and Enajon ranges are excellent choices, and the Musashi company makes high quality amino acids. These companies provide product without excessive 'filler' to make the pill or powder look bulkier and more impressive. Other additives are also kept to a minimum and all qualify for accreditation under the guidelines set by the Therapeutic Goods Administration. When you start using these preparations, you are getting science on your side.

TEAM WORK

Antioxidants and amino acids cover the essentials. The antioxidants provide protection and the amino acids provide performance. In combination, they make the A team. They work well together. They do not clash or diminish their effects when in your bloodstream simultaneously. This cannot be said for all other supplements. However, the benefits of other supplements may be real. There are thousands of supplement devotees who swear that they feel better and perform better when regularly taking other concoctions. But if you start taking everything that sounds logical and has high profile people backing the story, you'll end up rattling when you walk. (You'll have to walk because with all the money you're spending, you won't be able to afford to drive any longer!)

If you are determined to take something outside the amino acid and antioxidant families of vitamins A, C and E, find out what the active ingredients in each preparation are. Ask how they are manufactured, and most importantly, how the purported benefits occur. What else is used to give bulk to the powder, pill or liquid? What ingredients are affected by the use-by date? What scientific trials have been conducted? Have any of the testimonials provided by athletes and other role models been paid for? Importantly, does the supplement have approval under the Therapeutic Goods Administration guidelines? Just because you swallow the pill, doesn't mean you have to swallow the whole story.

Don't expect too much and put in too little. Drinking a sports drink instead of a soft drink won't make you a better athlete. Taking vitamin B before you drink a dozen beers won't prevent the alcoholic damage to your brain cells and liver. Popping a few antioxidants and amino acids will certainly help, but they are not a magic formula.

Eating well enough to score your 12 points each day is definitely the way to go.

MAKING THE MOST OF YOUR DOSE
Be aware of the importance of the method you use to take your supplements. Tablets and capsules generally have the problem of what is called 'bio-availability': if you take

1 gram of a substance, you will not absorb the complete 1 gram; a percentage will be metabolised and lost as the liver is absorbing it. It's preferable to take supplements in pure powder form if possible. While this method may be less palatable, it will maximise bio-availability and minimise metabolic losses. Ask yourself, am I taking these vitamins and amino acids because they taste nice, or am I using these products to provide a specific benefit?

Most importantly, don't take your supplements all year as a matter of routine. Your body is the world adjustment champion. We have an incredible ability to accommodate change. We can get used to eating half as much or twice as much food. We can get used to heat, cold, midnight sun or days of darkness. Your body can develop a tolerance to alcohol if you are a drinker (even though the body is still suffering damage); it can develop a tolerance to pain if you are a chronic sufferer. We can adjust to all kinds of deprivation and excess, and nutritional supplements are no different. It's true that some supplements take up to 3 months to reach full effectiveness, though in the longer term their impact will diminish if you just take them and take them and take them.

> The more we take supplements, the less effective they are! You won't be told this on the label of your bottle of vitamins, but you will develop a tolerance to the supplements you take if you take them all the time. Don't do this. I favour a simple system of three months on and one month off. It's easy to remember when you work by a calendar and the cost is less than when you take the vitamins every day, every month, all year.

If you find yourself with a sore throat or the sniffles during one of your 'off' months, simply swallow a couple of cloves of garlic, get some chilli down any way you can and go back on your supplements, especially vitamin C, for the next two days. Then return to your normal system of three months on, one month off.

You don't receive Every Day Counts points by taking supplements; you are, however, adding another asset to your health register, another boost to your immune system and a boost to your long-term health and vitality.

THE SEDUCTION OF STEROIDS

If you think the message about the dangers of anabolic steroid usage has been effective, think again. In his book, *Mind, Body and Sport*, John Douillard reported a study in which 100 aspiring athletes were asked the question: 'If you could take a pill which would guarantee that you would win the Gold Medal at the next Olympics and would also kill you within a year, would you take that pill?' The response was astounding. Well over half of the athletes would have taken that lethal pill. They would swap their life for their goal.

We shouldn't be surprised at the depth of the desire some athletes have to succeed, because taking lethal pills and injections is exactly what thousands continue to do every day across the country in an effort to reach the top, or just to feel better about themselves.

What about the rest of us? We may not be elite athletes, but we can still be tempted, especially if we are ignorant of the nature of steroids, and their dangerous side-effects.

The word *steroid* refers to naturally occurring hormones in the body, which are chemically copied with the aim of enhancing strength and performance. The term *anabolic* means *to build* or *rebuild*. Anabolic steroids assist tissues to repair themselves and help to restore energy levels and protein reserves. We all produce natural anabolic steroids. In women the major natural sex hormones or steroid hormones are estrogen and progesterone. Males naturally produce the potent anabolic steroid, testosterone. Women also produce testosterone, but only in small quantities, usually less than 10% of that of male testosterone production.

There are some legitimate uses for anabolic steroids. These include treatment for severe malnutrition and muscle wasting, and they have also been prescribed for sufferers of osteoporosis and bone fractures.

To be honest, we must admit that steroids work very effectively. In the short term, if you train hard with weights while you are taking steroids, you will gain in muscle size. Make no mistake, they work. That's why so many people are tempted to take them. They can do great things. Weak-minded people think that if you look stronger on the outside you will be stronger on the inside as a result.

Beware! There are other effects, like the masculinisation of many of the receptor tissues that are effected by steroids. Females who use anabolic steroids over a prolonged period often display obvious signs of maleness. The table below shows both the anabolic and androgenic, or secondary, effects of steroids use.

Anabolic effects	Androgenic and side effects
increased skeletal muscle mass	increased density and pattern of pubic hair
increased organ mass	irreversible deepening of voice
increased blood haemoglobin	increased sexual desire
increased red blood cell mass	increased blood pressure
increased calcium in bones	increased fluid retention
increased nitrogen retention	irreversible increase in facial hair

increased protein synthesis	scalp hair loss
	cystic acne
	decreased breast size, clitoral enlargement and menstrual irregularities in women

There are also separate side-effects. Consider these:

- liver function abnormalities
- hepatitis
- benign and malignant liver tumours
- prostrate cancer
- testicular atrophy
- increased cholesterol leading to increased risk of heart disease
- impaired immunity
- sterility
- premature death.

In the late seventies I was a young footballer trying to make a name in what was then the VFL. A team-mate and I were considered underweight and we were offered steroids to help bulk us up quickly. I ducked for cover, but my team-mate went for it. Within a month his voice had changed and he was physically lashing out at people at the drop of a hat. This caused problems with his girlfriend and it didn't help when he could no longer perform for her in other areas! He did get bigger and stronger, but he kept straining muscles and he couldn't control his aggression when he eventually did make it on to the field. The steroids really altered his psyche and his career petered out before it ever really got started. It was tragic at the time and it's had a negative impact on his life ever since.

Please ask yourself this question. If you use or are planning to use steroids, what is it that you are trying to change? Just your performance, or you as a person? If you 'get on the gear' you will be changing yourself forever. Consider these psychological shifts directly attributable to steroid usage:

- increased desire to train
- increased aggressive behaviour
- increased hostility
- increased pain tolerance
- increased evidence of mood swings.

Steroids may give you a better body in the short term but they could ruin you as a person, both physically and emotionally. Think of the burden of a prematurely decaying body, a guilty conscience from the 'cheat complex,' the knowledge that you have been dishonest, and a disturbed mindset complete with too much aggression and unstable moods. This is a foolproof plan to ruin your life.

It is estimated that at least 50% and as many as 90% of steroid users become addicted to the drug. The state of uncontrollable behaviour change, known as 'roid rage,' has been linked to actual documented cases of domestic violence and other forms of aggression, including suicide and homicide.

Life is too good to destroy and there are no guarantees of living happily ever after, even with a gold medal around your neck. Anabolic steroids are illegal, unnatural, life-shortening and life-threatening. Many athletes have died as a direct result of both short- and long-term steroid use. Steroids disturb the fine natural balance of our physiology and our psychology. While some people have achieved greater sporting success as a result of using anabolic steroids, none has lived a happier life through resorting to steroids, and almost all regret their usage.

What do I do now?

It's a good time now to introduce some of the Every Day Counts principles into your daily life. While I won't be asking you to implement the full system for a couple of weeks, it would be great if you could start getting in some practice.

1 Be aware of the fat content, in grams, of the foods you eat during the course of the day.
2 Use the tables in Appendix 2 to learn the fat content, in grams, of some of your favourite foods.
3 Start keeping a mental total of the amounts of fat, in grams, you are eating during the course of the day.
4 Begin allocating scores to each food choice you make. Keep a mental or written tally of your positive (+1), neutral (0) and negative (−1) choices during the course of the day.
5 Aim at scoring a total of 12 food points over the course of the day.
6 Consider beginning a regular intake of antioxidants and amino acids.

TRAINING TO KEEP WELL

*'Anyone engaged in mathematics or other
intellectual pursuits should also take part in some
form of physical training.'*

PLATO

READY FOR ACTION?

The exercise message has been around since Plato's time
and yet 2000 years later most of us are still struggling to
find a way to do anything about it. Regular exercise is like
buying a dollar for 50 cents: exercise pays dividends for a
lifetime. Thinking about it is not enough; you have to do
something about it.

There is a story about an old priest being posted to a
country town. He made an immediate impact when he
delivered a sensational first sermon. His message was so
strong that the congregation broke into spontaneous
applause after he had finished. It was the first time in
anyone's memory that the town's people had actually
clapped a homily.

The old priest talked about commonsense and basic
values. He spoke about honesty, integrity and helping
those in the community who needed support. He advised

parents that time spent with their children would never be wasted. He invited people to volunteer for charitable works and he encouraged everyone to treat others as they would like to be treated themselves. Everyone agreed that what he had to say made a lot of sense. There were heads nodding everywhere and not one person left early. He was articulate, passionate and inspiring.

The priest was very busy and visible around town that first week as he began to learn about his new parish and the people who lived in it. He didn't like what he saw. In the meantime, word spread quickly about the new preacher and the following week the church was filled to overflowing. To the surprise of many, the old priest delivered exactly the same sermon. Even though most people had heard it word for word only 7 days earlier, his delivery and sincerity again impressed them. The priest obviously meant every word he said.

Over the course of the next month the priest continued with this identical sermon, each and every Sunday. Attendances stopped growing and then even began to fall away alarmingly. The churchgoers just couldn't understand why he wasn't changing the topic. Eventually, after his sixth straight week of delivering the same sermon, the priest broke tradition by asking if there were any questions. After an uneasy silence, a well-known parishioner and community leader stood and tentatively began, 'Father, we've all been greatly impressed with what you have said over the past 6 weeks. But don't you think after all this time, it would be good for you to change what you're saying?'

The old priest had found the majority of his flock to be more Christian in name than in nature. He had been disappointed to see people cutting each other off just to get a better spot in the car park or smiling at someone on the way into church and then slandering them on the way out. He simply replied: 'My son, I'll be happy to change what I'm doing as soon as you do!'

> The moral of the story is that just because we hear a good suggestion, and agree that we should do something about it, doesn't mean that we will. Exercise is the ultimate case of 'good in theory, hard in practice'. We need a system to follow.

Over the 20 centuries since Plato first promoted the virtues of regular exercise, the message has been more often repeated than it has been heeded. We're still spruiking Plato's advice, and we've never been more in need of it than we are today.

EXERCISE EXCUSES

People have some weird and wonderful ideas about exercise and some imaginative excuses for not exercising. My favourite is the 'heartbeat theory'. I first heard about this theory from one of the great exercise avoiders of all time, an accountant friend of mine named Greg. A few years ago, Greg's company was sponsoring morning exercise sessions and the managers were encouraged to attend.

Greg is a very resourceful guy and he made it his mission in life to avoid the sessions. He told me that he was really a masochist who liked nothing better than to get out of bed every morning at six and run 10 kilometres. He claimed that was the only reason he religiously stayed in bed until eight. He told me that he was punishing himself by staying in bed longer.

He then claimed that he was already doing 40 kilometres each week, but he admitted under cross-examination that 38 of them were in his car. This guy would do anything short of contracting an infectious disease to avoid exercise. To his mind, exercise really was the plague. Greg was fooling no one and so he knew that the usual excuses of 'no time' or 'no energy' wouldn't get him out of the sessions. Greg decided to come up with something original.

Next he tried the receding hair theory. I was taking the early morning classes at the time and because my hair was receding, Greg figured there must be a connection. He assumed that if you exercise too often you would start to lose your hair. I think Greg's definition of working out too often was once a year!

After I'd introduced him to a few people who still had plenty of hair 'on top' even though they had been working out for years, he turned to his sexual inadequacy theory. This one goes that if you are a male, the fitter you are, the more quickly you reach climax during sex. I wasn't keen to delve into Greg's private life too closely, especially because Greg's wife, Karen, was within earshot at the time he was explaining what he called his 'wham-bam-sorry mam' theory. Karen quickly solved that dilemma when she told Greg that he 'couldn't get much worse, so a bit of exercise might actually improve his stamina'. Greg also admitted that whenever his doctor asked him about sex, he would always answer 'infrequently' so his doctor would never be sure whether he meant his answer as one word or two!

This left Greg desperate and with only one excuse left in his bag of tricks. If he wanted to avoid getting out of bed an hour earlier three times per week, it needed to be good. That's when he finally came up with his pièce de résistance, the infamous 'heartbeat theory'. According to Greg's heartbeat theory, we are all born with a certain number of available heartbeats. Once you use up these heartbeats, it's all over. Greg was determined to save as many heartbeats as he could. He was convinced that he was doing himself a favour by resting and conserving each precious beat of his heart. He was from the school of thinking that says why walk when you can drive, and that there is no point in picking up a weight when you are just going to have to put it down again.

Greg was a believer in early to bed and late to rise and he was the classic remote control addict. He would be sure to take the motorised walkway at the airport instead of walking from the gate lounge to collect his baggage. Sure he'd been sitting on the plane for hours, but why waste energy, right? His idea of a workout was to fill up the bath, take up the plug and fight the current. He didn't want to hear that exercise strengthens your heart. He didn't care that with each beat, more blood would be pushed around the body. 'Mine beats just fine the way it is,' he said, 'so why should I try to change it. Why run around the block when I'm already here?'

He was unimpressed that the main reason we need blood is to carry oxygen. Oxygen is what our muscles and our brain need for survival. Oxygen is used to break food down into energy so our muscles can pull our bones around. He didn't care that a fit person with a strong heart has a far greater capacity to bring in fresh oxygen and get rid of the stale, oxygen-depleted air laden with carbon dioxide. 'All that oxygen would just make me light-headed. If I need more oxygen I can drive up a mountain,' Greg would say. I should have explained to Greg that it is actually the other way around: there is less and less oxygen the higher you go. However, I thought it would be prudent to let the oxygen and altitude dilemma go and concentrate on attacking Greg's heartbeat theory.

HOW MANY HEARTBEATS?

What Greg needed to know was that people who exercise have lower resting heart rates. People who are fit can have resting heart rates of less than 50 beats per minute. Elite footballers have resting heart rates as low as 40 beats per minute or even less.

A resting heart rate of 50 beats per minute will serve as an example. The average adult resting heart rate is around 72 beats per minute. Greg's resting rate was 75 beats per minute. The fit person's heart is beating 25 times less than Greg's every minute of its life. Therefore it is 'saving' 25 beats every minute compared to Greg's. It's doing the same work with less effort. (Of course, Greg argued, 'Yes, but he uses up those beats big time whenever he exercises, so he's worse off.')

When you do the figures the fit person saving 25 beats every minute saves 1500 beats every hour and 43 200 beats every day. When a fit person trains, his or her heart rate normally sits around 150 beats per minute for about an hour. The most a person who trains regularly will 'use' is an additional 6000 beats per day (60 mins × 100 beats per minute).

The total equation shows that you save over 43 000 beats every day by having a lower resting heart rate. Even when you have trained that day, the net saving is 37 000 heartbeats. This has to be an attractive investment: invest 6000 for a 37 000 return. I wish my superannuation fund could do that. Exercise really is better than a 'dollar for 50 cents' investment. I thought this might appeal to someone with Greg's background in accounting and finance, I hoped that I finally had him convinced when I calculated that a saving of 37 000 heartbeats each day meant that your heart was going to be beating 13.5 million times less each year! That's not a bad cost-benefit analysis. Greg was surprised and impressed and to everyone's astonishment he even began coming to the morning sessions!

Unfortunately, he soon dropped out when he started finding a few strands of hair on his comb. Oh well, you can't win them all, but I haven't given up on Greg yet! He's walking most mornings and he takes his pulse rate every morning. The walking sessions have reduced his resting heart rate from 75 beats per minute to 63 beats per minute. Greg calls it his balanced approach. He says he's 'saving heartbeats and hair at the same time'.

GETTING THE GET-UP-AND-GO TO GET UP AND GO

Even though we're all aware of some of the benefits of regular exercise, you may, like Greg, be pleasantly surprised by some of the great things exercise can do for us.

- *Regular exercise improves cardiovascular efficiency.* This means your lungs take in more oxygen and transfer it more easily into the bloodstream. The circulatory system carries the oxygen more easily to the muscles and brain. Everything we do takes a lot less effort.

- *Exercise increases what is called stroke volume.* The heart is a muscle and it increases in size and strength as a response to regular training. A larger, stronger heart pumps out more blood with each beat, both at rest and when under exertion. You have more power when you need it and your heart doesn't have to work as hard as it used to. (So much for Greg's heart-beat theory.)

- *Exercise lowers your resting heart rate.* Because the heart pumps more blood with each beat, when at rest, it doesn't have to beat as often.

- *Exercise acts as a waste disposal system.* If we never breathe deeply, a 'plug' of carbon dioxide stays in our lungs throughout the day. It just goes up and down inside our windpipe as we take small, shallow breaths. When we exercise, our deeper exhalations directly eliminate this waste. When we sweat, we also get rid of the by-products of our metabolic processes and digestion. This happens through moisture in our breath and through the pores of our skin.

- *Exercise relaxes our muscles.* We think of tension as being an emotional state when in reality it's also a physical state. Muscles get tight and tense and need exercise or massage to help counter small nodes of tension that build up around them. Exercise stretches and increases the temperature of muscles. As they become more malleable they change shape with all the bending, straightening and rotation involved in exercise. These nodes of tension are washed back into the bloodstream and are outed either through breathing or when we go to the toilet.

- *Exercise improves muscle tone.* Muscle tone is how ready and willing your muscles are to contract. If you are constantly working your muscles, they will stay partially contracted all of the time. That's why they feel firmer to the touch. The more muscle fibres you contract, the firmer your muscles feel.

  This is also one of the reasons why regular exercise increases metabolism and makes it easier to maintain your ideal weight. It takes energy to keep these muscle fibres contracted. If you never exercise, your muscles get used to the constant state of relaxation and so they don't bother staying contracted at all. That's why untrained muscles feel loose and soft to the touch. Your resting metabolic rate will be slower than that of someone who exercises regularly. It also makes it harder to maintain your ideal weight when you don't exercise.

- *Exercise also fulfils an intrinsic human need.* It is one of the necessities of life. We need to eat and keep warm and we have strong natural desires to be loved, make love and gain acceptance in our lives. Your body needs to exercise. All animals have this need and we are no different. Deprivation of any of our primal needs can cause emotional and physical problems.
- *Exercise can also help reduce blood pressure, headaches, fluid retention and digestive problems.*

For many people exercise declines with age. It starts in childhood as a natural instinct to play, changes in adolescence to a way to spend some time, and eventually fades away to something there is no time for as busy adults. If you suppress your urge to exercise long enough it will become dormant in adulthood. It's just what happens to us. As kids we just play, as teenagers we play sport and as adults we play the markets. Exercise is relegated to the 'when I get time' category, the same category that still has last year's tax return waiting for attention.

EXERCISE NOT 'EXERLIES'

The previous chapter revealed that your first step to healthy living was to control your fat intake so that you will score 12 food points each day and maintain your fat intake between 40 and 50 grams.

Your second step to finding the Health Zone is to 'Raise a sweat through exercise on 4 out of every 7 days'.

An hour of gentle exercise on these days will score you the 4 points you need within our Every Day Counts system.

The exercise guidelines and programs set out in this chapter will not turn you into an athlete. The only race they are designed to prepare you for is the human race. In Chapter 10 we will look at fitness training as a separate area. Right now your focus is to learn how exercise can count every day.

In the Every Day Counts system, I am asking you to exercise on 4 days out of every 7. A system of 'day on, day off' works well if you think on a fortnightly basis. Just make sure that you train on successive days some time during the second week of each fortnight. This ensures you keep with your schedule of 4 exercise days each week. Just to make sure you understand what I mean, this is how that system works.

E stands for Exercise day and R stands for Rest day.

Day	1	2	3	4	5	6	7	8	9	10	11	12	13	14
	E	R	E	R	E	R	E	E	R	E	R	E	R	E

Alternatively, you may choose to train on 2 consecutive days and then have a rest day. You can even have 2 rest days in a row. Two consecutive days of rest is the maximum you should allow yourself. You will begin to lose many training benefits after 48 hours of continuous inactivity, so watch out! Here is an example of this system.

Day	1	2	3	4	5	6	7
	E	E	R	E	E	R	R

The most important thing to do is keep your exercise regular and average those 4 sessions each week.

On the 4 days that you do exercise, your overall Every Day Counts target is 20 points (12 food points + 4 exercise points +

4 pressure points). On the 3 rest days each week, your target is
16 points (12 food points + 4 pressure points).

You score 1 exercise point for each 15 consecutive minutes
of activity. A workout of 1 hour will give you the 4 points you're
aiming at for that day (4×15 mins = 4×1 points = 4 points).

Equally, 4 separate workouts of 15 minutes would
also enable you to reach your target for that day, though
in reality this would be impractical for most people. Put
the time together at your own discretion, though you
need those 60 training minutes on 4 of the 7 days in
each week.

It's a good idea to give yourself some time to build up
to this level of 1 hour of exercise on 4 out of every 7 days.
The best approach is to spend 2 weeks phasing yourself
into the program and getting used to counting food,
exercise and pressure points.

The system actually allows you to earn up to 6 exercise
points on any single day. Ninety minutes of exercise is
required to achieve 6 exercise points. This flexibility is
designed to help you balance out a day where you don't
eat well enough to accumulate 12 food points or when
you don't manage to schedule enough relaxation or stress
management time to achieve 4 stress points. A little give
and take between the three vital areas is what living in
the Health Zone is all about. Every Day Counts allows
you to keep balance by using one of the three areas to
boost up another.

You may choose to exercise even longer than 90
minutes, though this will never score you additional points
on any day. You cannot use exercise points to contribute
toward your target on non-exercise days. The system
provides you with some leeway, not loopholes. As the
tightrope walkers say, 'It's all a matter of balance.'

People often ask me, 'What is the best type of exercise to do?' They may have seen the latest exercise machine advertised on television. Inevitably they will want to know whether this machine works any better or faster than others they have already tried and discarded. The answer is they work if you use them.

The biomechanical advantage of one machine over another is very minor. The emphasis is on the word 'use'. You know that saying, 'Use it or lose it'? My saying is 'Sweat or regret'! No machine can work if you leave it in the closet. The type of exercise is very much secondary to the fact that you are doing something on a regular basis. In Chapter 10 we will look at fitness and specific conditioning. At the moment we are interested in wellness. To protect your health, it's the regularity of exercise rather than the type of exercise that is the imperative. In our Every Day Counts system, all exercise is equal and it all counts as 1 point for 15 minutes invested.

WHAT'S HOT AND WHAT'S NOT

So what counts as exercise and what doesn't? The definition of exercise is very simple: When you are moving more than you are resting, it qualifies as exercise. When you are resting more than you are moving, it doesn't qualify. Regular movement is the key. This doesn't mean you could walk for 8 minutes and then rest for 7 minutes and still have your 15-minute session qualify for 1 exercise point. It means that you have to keep moving most of the time. Rest periods of up to 60 seconds are acceptable in the normal course of recovering between jogs, collecting tennis balls, waiting between badminton rallies, resting between sets of exercises or waiting between laps of the pool. If you are passive for more than a minute at a time, it doesn't score.

Some people are very active at work and think they get all the exercise they need that way. Unfortunately for them, even though they may move around a lot, they are also usually forced to continually stop to check a machine, fix a problem, answer a phone call or talk to a colleague. In physical terms this means rest, a reduction in heart and breathing rates. It also means an interruption to the continual movement needed to make the exercise worthwhile and score exercise points. This restriction even applies to people who cover what seems like kilometres as part of their job and are legitimately tired at the end of the day. Even when you are on your feet almost all day, your work time will not automatically score exercise points. If you have some flexibility in your work, you may be able to schedule times when you do keep moving for at least 15 minutes without interruption. It would be a great asset if you could combine work and exercise. This applies to supervisors, builders and other tradespeople, retailers, factory managers, council workers, parking officers and many others.

Even if exercise is the last thing you feel like doing outside work hours, it's the only way to get the extra energy you're looking for. When you invest some energy you'll get a lot more back in return. Exercise gently before or after work and remember to keep the movement continual.

Here are some examples of activities that are worth 1 Every Day Counts point for every 15-minute segment: aerobic classes, badminton, basketball, bushwalking, calisthenics, circuit training, cycling, dancing, digging, football, gardening (as long as you are mowing, weeding, hoeing or raking more than you are stationary), handball, hockey, jogging, netball, pump classes, roller blading, running, soccer, squash, sweeping, swimming, tennis (make sure you retrieve the balls as quickly as you can), walking and weight training (no more than 1 minute rest between sets).

Here are some examples of activities that fail to qualify: lawn bowls, meditation, tai chi, ten pin bowling, weight training (if you have more than 1 minute between sets) and yoga. Some of these activities qualify as pressure activities rather than as exercise.

Other activities can work for you if you limit the rest periods, though they don't qualify automatically. Tennis is a classic example. If you serve your share of double faults and your opponent either hits winners or out balls on the first return, you can spend a lot of passive time while the balls are collected or you wait for your opponent to get ready for the next rally. Baseball, cricket, croquet and gymnastics also fit into this category.

Playing golf on foot by yourself or with one partner certainly qualifies because you will be walking or hitting more often than you are waiting for your turn. If you are in a 4-ball, it's likely that you will be waiting and resting too often to qualify. However, when you play 18 holes on foot you actually walk about 7 kilometres. This is a great and worthwhile thing to do and is enough to earn your exercise points for that day.

All activity qualifies as long as you make sure you keep moving more than you are resting over a 15-minute period and without any individual rest periods exceeding 60 seconds. Our criteria are based on continuity, not intensity. Keep moving and you will tally up the exercise points you need very easily.

WARMING TO THE TASK

Whatever sport or exercises you choose, before you start please warm up. A proper warm up reduces muscle soreness. When we exercise, we place our bodies under greater demands than when we are resting or performing everyday activities. If your body is not prepared adequately, it will suffer.

During the initial phase of any exercise session there is an increased demand for oxygen, and accelerated blood flow. Warming up readies the body for this overload. If you suddenly started sprinting up the nearest hill, your body would need to quickly send extra blood to the working muscles, especially the quadriceps and calf muscles of your legs. With this rush of blood towards the lower half of your body, the flow of blood to the top half must be reduced. There is only so much to go around. Our bodies can handle this as long as we allow some adjustment time. Warming up provides this. If you don't, do it, you'll be too dizzy to enjoy the view from the top of that hill you just sprinted up.

Warming up increases blood flow not just to, but through, the muscles. As blood vessels dilate, there is an increase in the local temperature of the muscle and the oxygen supply. You will feel this gradual warming up of your body as you start to sweat. Your breathing will also be faster and deeper.

Warming up decreases viscosity in the muscles. This means that they contract and relax more quickly. Your body will begin to feel a lot looser and more supple. Warming up increases the speed and force of muscle contractions. Your movements are quicker and reaction times faster when you have warmed up.

Don't fall for the temptation of skimping on your warm up or warm down. Missing the warm up phase will only make it harder for your cardiovascular system to adjust to the steady state you are trying to maintain. When you don't warm up, your heart rate response may become erratic and unpredictable. It's common to experience unwanted highs and lows in heart rates during the early phase of exercise when the warm up has been insufficient. These are the very things you are trying to avoid.

Ultimately you'll end up burning less kilojoules trying to save time, so it won't be a saving at all. When this phenomenon was called 'getting your second wind' it was considered to be an 'old wives tale'. Now we know just how real and important it is and the old wives have been proven right once again.

Warming up has been compared to foreplay. It's tempting to go straight to what comes later, but when you take the time, the entire experience is always more enjoyable!

Now for the warning. Exercise can kill, but nowhere near as often as the lack of it. Cases of exercise-induced heart attacks are rare but well publicised. They often deter potential exercisers from ever reintroducing activity into their lives. These cases can provide a very convenient and comfortable excuse for us not to exercise. It is the lifestyle of abuse and neglect that causes heart disease: controlled exercise will help prevent it!

Sure, if you have been hardening your arteries for 20 years and you suddenly try to run 10 kilometres at Olympic qualifying pace then you're asking for trouble. Let commonsense prevail. If you're over 35, or have led a sedentary life for the last five years, have a medical check up before you start. After all, the aim of your program is to improve your lifestyle and free yourself from worry about your health. It's going to be hard to do this if every time you work out it's in the back of your mind that you might keel over! Start out with a clear mind, not just new shorts. Take a medical!

DETERMINING YOUR HEART RATE TARGET

Hopefully, you are now asking yourself questions like, 'What should I actually do to earn my exercise points?' and 'How hard should I push myself?' There are some guidelines to follow.

We know that to score exercise points the only prerequisite is to ensure that you are active more than you are resting. This is all you really need. However, if you are the type of person who would like to be more specific about how intense your exercise should be, then determining your heart rate target is vital!

The table below provides you with both a heart rate training range as well as a specific heart rate target number to aim at. You will achieve an effective workout when your heart rate is somewhere between the two nominated training range figures while you are exercising. The ideal is to exercise as close as possible to your specific heart rate target number.

Age	Activity level	Perceived exertion	Heart rate range	Target number
20	low	medium	140–155	147
	moderate	medium	140–160	150
	high	medium	145–165	155
30	low	medium	130–145	137
	moderate	medium	130–150	140
	high	medium	135–155	145
40	low	medium	120–135	127
	moderate	medium	120–140	130
	high	medium	125–145	135
50	low	medium	110–125	117
	moderate	medium	110–130	120
	high	medium	115–135	125
60+	low	medium	100–115	107
	moderate	medium	100–120	110
	high	medium	105–125	115

The table is designed to help you work out what your own heart rate target range and heart rate target number will be. In this table, the *Activity level* column relates to your current level of activity. 'High' means you are already exercising four or more times each week, 'moderate' relates to someone who exercises two or three times each week, while 'low' describes someone who trains no more than once each week. The *Perceived exertion* column recommends that you should aim at a moderate or 'medium' level of intensity during your workouts. This equates to you subjectively rating your workouts as being 6 out of 10 on a scale of difficulty.

Every Day Counts requires only that your exercise is consistent and continual for at least 15 minutes, without any rest period exceeding 60 seconds. Using target heart rates controls the next dimension: intensity. Your *Heart rate range* column and your specific *Target number* column guide the intensity. Manipulate your workout so that you are as close as possible to your actual target heart rate number. It's very important that you at least stay within your target range. When you do this you will enjoy a successful and safe workout.

Any activity that has more movement time than rest time will elevate your pulse rate, though some types of training are more effective than others in maintaining your heart rate at the required level. Exercise will be ineffective if your heart rate keeps rising above and dipping below the upper and lower thresholds of your training range.

One way of achieving this heart rate stability is through the use of indoor aerobic equipment like a stationary bike, rower or treadmill. There are many advantages and the convenience factor is the most important. You can work out in your own home and you don't have to brave the early morning elements, which can be less than inviting in the middle of winter when it's dark, cold and lonely.

Cycling, rowing, walking and running are the most effective forms of exercise when you are trying to maintain a narrow heart rate range. This is because there are very few variables (except for hills) to upset your rhythm and make your heart rate jump up or drop down.

There are dozens of exercise strategies that will work for you. Perhaps you could start your day with a 60-minute workout to score 4 exercise points. The latest fitness research has shown that we keep burning kilojoules for hours after an early morning workout. The keys are to exercise before your first meal of the day and to keep your pulse rate as close as possible to your specific target point. If you train for 60 minutes prior to breakfast on each of your exercise days, you will burn kilojoules not only for the 60 minutes you are working out, but you'll be burning energy for up to another 4 hours. That's 4 hours of free kilojoules burning in excess of what you would achieve at rest.

The longer you maintain this habit, the more permanent this boost to your basal metabolic rate will be. It all adds up to the most efficient time of the day to train. Time efficiency is also a consideration. You only need to get out of bed 60 minutes earlier than normal to achieve a morning workout. Jogging, cycling, walking and rowing are simple and safe so you can warm up while you wake up.

You should aim to reach your target heart rate by the start of the sixth minute of your morning workout. You then hold this target rate for the next 48 minutes. After this, take 6 minutes to slow down and gradually lower your heart rate back toward your normal resting level. That's 60 minutes well spent. Following this, it's into the shower and on to breakfast knowing that your exercise points for the day are already half achieved. If you don't have time, you could train for 30 minutes and before breakfast achieve 2 exercise points for the day. You'll enjoy your muesli all the more knowing that your metabolism will remain elevated right through until lunchtime. It's a good feeling.

Many indoor machines like bikes and rowers have 'heart rate control options'. This allows you to input your desired heart rate at the beginning of your workout. The machine then monitors and adjusts the level of resistance so that you not only stay within a target range; you stay right on your specific heart rate target number. If your heart rate gets too high, the machine makes it easier for you to pedal or pull. If your heart rate is too low, the machine makes you work harder. This maximises the efficiency of your workout and the number of kilojoules you expend. It all adds up to a simple, convenient, time-efficient and safe way to train.

If you are using an exercise bike, the most efficient riding position is when you extend your legs fully on each pedal downstroke. Don't be tempted to use a lower seat position in the hope that you will burn more energy because it's harder work when you can't straighten your legs. This will only lead to problems with your hamstring muscles and lower back. Lift the seat to a comfortably high position.

What do I do now?
You can't buy exercise. There is no exercise pill. Personal trainers are great but even they can't sweat for you. Please, give it a try. Let's look at some specific workout ideas to help get you started and get you counting.

6

WORKOUT FOR POINTS

*'The best plan is only a plan, that is good intentions,
until it degenerates into work.'*

DRUCKER

WALK YOUR WAY TO POINTS

Exercise science has shown us that with every step we run, we land with a force equivalent to three or four times our body weight. This force is transmitted into our feet, up through our legs into our pelvis and lower back. If you are well conditioned and accustomed to running, you will readily absorb these forces as you sustain or improve your present fitness level. The evidence continues to mount, however, that when it comes to beginners embarking on the road or track to a healthier body, running may have to wait.

A deconditioned person's musculoskeletal system may lack the shock absorption capability to deal with the triple body weight shocks of each running step. The problem is made worse if the new runner is overweight, a condition that is common and often the very reason people have decided to begin or return to regular activity.

When commencing a walking program, the three big questions are: How fast? How far? How often?

Casey Meyers, in his book *Walking*, reported on a 1991 study conducted by Dr John Duncan that compared the efficiency of three walking speeds: 12 minutes per kilometre (5 kilometres per hour), 9 minutes per kilometre (6.6 kilometres per hour) and 7 minutes per kilometre (8.5 kilometres per hour). The subjects were all previously inactive women and the overwhelming motivation was weight loss and weight control. The results were clear. Those walking at the quicker pace of 7 minutes per kilometre used much more energy than the other groups. All groups covered 5 kilometres, 5 times per week. The quicker group spent 3 hours of actual walking time per week compared to 5 hours per week for the slowest group, the 12 minutes per kilometre group.

Even though they were exercising for 2 hours less per week, the group that walked fastest expended 2500 more kilojoules than the slowest group. Over a 12-month period, when walking 5 kilometres, 5 times per week this extrapolates to an additional energy burn of over 128 000 kilojoules and a further weight loss of 4 kilograms. That's 4 less kilograms you'll have to carry around. This all comes from walking a bit faster.

It is clear that it is most efficient to walk as fast as you comfortably can: 7–8 minutes per kilometre should be your goal. Any faster than that is almost a run. Slower speeds are still worthwhile, but it will take longer to get the same result, especially if you are managing your weight.

Now let's find out what's a good speed for you. If you are just starting out, try this. For your first week, walk 2.5 kilometres, 4 times per week at an intensity that you find comfortable. This is likely to be in the 10–12 minutes per kilometre range so you will be actually walking for between 25 and 30 minutes. You will score 2 exercise points for each workout, although this is secondary at the moment. Don't be too concerned with your speed or your points at this stage, just try to enjoy being out there! It's not a worry that you won't score the 4 exercise points. We will build up to this during the recommended 2-week transition period.

During week 2, increase your speed without increasing your distance. Stay at 4 sessions of 2.5 kilometres each time. Gradually increase your speed until you can maintain 7–8 minutes per kilometre pace for the distance. This means walking 2.5 kilometres in 20 minutes or less. Your rule of thumb is to never exceed a score of 7 out of 10 on your personal exertion scale. You should always leave something in reserve. This is paramount and takes precedence over your walking speed.

You may not reach these exact speeds. Everyone is different so work up to an appropriate speed for you. By the end of the week you will have a good idea of the fastest speed you can comfortably maintain for this distance. Stay with this speed. Up until now you will still have only been earning 1 or 2 Every Day Counts points per workout because you have been walking for less than half an hour. This is exactly what we've wanted up to this point. The next step is to start increasing the time factor.

From the start of week 3 progressively increase your walking time until you are completing 4 × 60-minute sessions every week. Try to stay at the desired intensity of 7–8 minutes per kilometre, or whatever your fastest comfortable walking speed turns out to be. In other words, try not to reduce your speed as you increase the distance. You will now be earning 4 score points every time you walk and you'll be burning a truckload of kilojoules.

You will find that you have to use your arms aggressively and lengthen your stride to sustain this 'fastest comfortable' tempo. There is no set rule as to how far your arms swing forward. This is dependent on the flexibility of your shoulder joint, the surrounding muscles, your posture and your co-ordination. It has to be natural. Go with your own style, but please remember the following technique points:

- You will not be able to sustain brisk walking pace by relying on your legs alone. If you keep your arms passive you will lack acceleration and the action of brisk walking will feel unnatural.
- When your arms are swinging aggressively forward, there may be a tendency to swing in and across your body. While it is natural for this to happen to some extent, excessive lateral movement will develop an inefficient and unbalanced side-to-side swaying action. It is to be avoided at all costs as it reduces speed and impairs balance and posture.

Many people are pleasantly surprised at how quickly they improve and just how much distance they can cover in 60 minutes. Walking is the best single exercise option we have to get back on the road to the Health Zone.

IF IT FITS LIKE A GLOVE . . . IT'S TOO TIGHT!

It is estimated that 90% of people wear their training shoes too tight. Recent US wear tests claim that this occurs for two reasons. Firstly, people don't have their feet measured, or haven't had their feet measured recently enough, and secondly, we relate glove fit to shoe fit. It's definitely a case of buyer beware: if the shoe fits, check again!

Gloves fit tight and firm, hence the saying, 'fits like a glove'. When it comes to our feet, however, we must allow for two additional factors: elongation and spread. Regardless of how well designed and made the shoe is, if it is too small and your foot is hanging over the platform, your feet will be cramped and impeded from carrying out their vital functions.

Always take your old shoes with you when you intend to purchase a new pair. You cannot assume that you are now the same size as you were even 12 months ago. You certainly can't assume that both feet are the same size. Almost 20% of people require at least a half size larger or smaller for one foot compared to the other. Your old shoes also tell a story about your gait, tread and degree of pronation (putting your foot into the prone position). Your shoe style should match your walking style.

How can you tell which pair is right for you by looking at the shoes? You can't! An expert fitter will instantly tell you whether you have a wide forefoot and narrow heel, a high instep, flat feet or a variety of other types.

Satisfy yourself that the expertise of the person at point of sale matches your requirements as a consumer. The major shoe companies and retail chains are making enormous efforts to increase the level of knowledge of their shoe fitters and this initiative is to be applauded without reservation. However, there are still times when the person serving you won't have all the answers you need.

Resist the temptation to buy on impulse, to buy according to fashion, or to buy according to your previous bias about which companies make the right shoes for your foot type and your sport or activity.

You must also be realistic about cross-training footwear. Cross-training shoes have a place in the market for people who may do some recreational running, play some volleyball and a game or two of tennis, but there always has to be a trade-off between lateral support, heel-toe cushioning and durability. You can't have it both ways. If you are serious about a specific activity, you will require a dedicated pair of shoes. You may require running shoes, court shoes *and* cross-trainers.

WORKING FROM HOME

When time is as precious as your need to incorporate regular exercise into your lifestyle and score exercise points, home training is an option to consider. It's surprising how little equipment you really need. You can get away with nothing other than two metres of rope, a chair and a set of light dumbbells. Of course the more equipment you have, the more you can do, but there are numerous exercises that require no equipment at all. One of the potential pitfalls in home-based training is that you tend to get distracted. Instead of exercising, it's easy to end up doing the dishes, answering the phone or reading the paper.

There is no doubt that circuit training is your best option because it keeps you moving. The advantage of circuit training is that it provides a structure for you to follow. There is a set order of exercises, a set period for each exercise and a set period of rest. You also have a definite start and finish to your workout. From a physical perspective, circuit training stresses both the muscular and cardio systems. You therefore benefit both in regard to your heart-lung fitness and improvements in your strength and tone. Every 15 minutes you spend circuit training at home will earn you 1 exercise point. A 60-minute circuit fulfils your 4-point exercise requirement for the day.

Here are 10 primary exercises that are straightforward to perform while providing whole-body benefits. They are outlined in the order in which you should do them in your home circuit.

1 *Skipping* Always start with an exercise that gets your entire body moving. This increases blood flow, warms muscles before they are asked to make specific and demanding moves and is a short cut to sweating. Sweating indicates that you are beginning to dissipate heat, a sure sign that your warm up is having the desired effect.

The best way for beginners to skip is to hop both feet at the same time over the rope. If you find this difficult, hold both ends of the rope in one hand and swing it by your side. Practise jumping both feet over the rope each time it is at its lowest point, until you master the basic art.

Your tempo should be slow. This is a warm up, not a world speed skipping record attempt. Try 20 and 30 skips per minute for 2 minutes, followed by a minute's rest and then another 2 minutes at 20 skips per minute. This will provide the warm up you need. You are on your way.

If you find skipping too hard, or too difficult to master, simply walk for 5 minutes to warm up.

Before you start the next exercise, please spend 3–5 minutes stretching. My best guess is that 9 out of 10 home exercisers skimp on stretching or don't stretch at all. The 3 minutes they think they are saving can't compensate for impaired performance and the hours of physio treatment they are likely to need as injury rehabilitation.

Every exercise should be done for 40 seconds and there is 40 seconds recovery between exercises.

2 *Shoulder press* You can do this exercise standing, but sitting with back support is preferable. Raise the dumbbells (or bricks or books) alternatively above your head until you reach full arm extension.

103

As one arm is lifting the other is lowering. Keep your head and hips as still as you can and concentrate on full, smooth moves instead of trying for a magic number of repetitions. Ten repetitions of the exercise done well are preferable to 20 done with dodgy technique.

3 *Triceps press* Hold one of the dumbbells, or whatever objects you are using for resistance, in both hands behind your head. Your elbows should be pointing forwards either side of your face (as if you are pushing your ears together with your arms). Keeping your elbows steady, straighten your arms by lifting the weight directly upward above your head. Slowly lower back to the starting position. Keep going until the time is up.

4 *Side stretches* Give your shoulders a rest by standing with your feet shoulder-width apart. Reach with your left arm downward along the left side of your body. Your right arm will naturally move upwards along the side of your rib cage. Reverse by moving your right arm downwards. Try to breathe evenly as you stretch to each side and avoid jerky movements. This exercise really works the hips and oblique abdominal.

5 *Inlocations* This is a movement of the shoulder joint controlled by the shoulder blades. Hold the dumbbells above your head, one in each hand. Lower both dumbbells forward in front of your face, then lift back 'up and over' until your arms are extending back as far as they can. The movement is like a back and forward windmill arm action and is an excellent shoulder and back strengthener. It's almost like a backstroke arm action except you swing both arms at the same time and you go over

and back rather than all the way around. You'll only need a light weight for this exercise.

6 *Abdominals* Sit ups are back in vogue. A full sit up starts with you lying on your back with your feet on the floor and your knees bent. Your feet are not held by a partner or braced under a bar or table. Without lifting your feet off the ground, raise your upper body until you can press your arms forward to touch your toes. Don't rest your hands on your head. The best positions are arms crossed in front of your chest or 'held in space' a couple of centimetres in front of your face.

7 *Shoulder turns* Hold each dumbbell directly above your shoulders with your elbows in front of you. This is like the position the weightlifters use before they press the bar above their heads. Twist your shoulders alternatively to the left and right as far as you find comfortable. Hold the dumbbells steady and you will gain benefits all the way from your hips to your shoulders.

8 *Angled push ups* Lean forward against a wall, or if you're ambitious support your weight by using a chair to lean all your weight against. Bend your arms so that your face moves closer to the wall or chair. Push outwards until your elbows are fully straightened. It's just like a normal push up except you are leaning against something instead of being flat on the ground. The further your feet are away from the wall or chair, the more resistance there will be in this exercise.

9 *Knee drives* Rest your sturdy chair against a wall. The chair must be able to support your total body weight easily. Step up onto the chair with one foot, step up with the other foot and as you do drive your

knee upward toward your chest. Step down one foot at a time and repeat. This is a fantastic exercise for keeping your behind in shape. Keep going until your time for this exercise has elapsed.

10 *Crunches* This is your second abdominal exercise. Lie on your back and elevate your legs. Keep a 90-degree knee and hip bend by resting your feet on a chair. Lift your trunk upwards until your elbows reach your knees. You can lightly grasp your ear lobes with your fingers to prevent pulling against your neck, or let your hands stay by your sides. Either way, breathe out as you rise up and inhale as you lower back.

It is important to control your circuit by time, not by a set number of repetitions. Please follow this schedule:

Time per exercise	40 seconds
Rest between exercises	40 seconds
Number of exercise stations	10

(Skipping is done slowly for 5 minutes as a warm up but the next time through the circuit it is treated like all other exercises and is performed for only 40 seconds.)

Number of times through circuit:

Beginner = 2 times = 30 minutes including stretch = 2 exercise points

Moderate = 3 times = 45 minutes including stretch = 3 exercise points.

Advanced = 4 times = 60 minutes including pre- and post-stretch = 4 exercise points.

Remember, there is no set number of repetitions per exercise. Work to time, not repetitions.

Home circuits really have some fantastic advantages. Equipment and costs are minimised, convenience is maximised, time efficiency can be no better and the quality of the workout can be extremely high. Home fitness won't always work if you thrive on social contact and external motivation, but if time and budget are tight, it could be the option for you.

LUNCH ON THE RUN

Here's a lunchtime workout of just 30 minutes duration. It's an aerobic entrée, muscles for main course, and a de-stressing dessert. It's the ultimate healthy lunch and it will earn you 2 exercise points every time it's on your menu.

There are three good reasons to work out at lunchtime. Any or all of these may apply to you:

1 If you lead a busy life, and family, social or other commitments prevent you from finding time for sufficient training sessions in the mornings or evenings, then lunchtime training must be an option for you.

2 If you are trying to control your weight, lunchtime workouts have the quadruple benefits of burning kilojoules, accelerating metabolic rates for the remainder of the afternoon, suppressing appetite and keeping you out of temptation's way while your workmates may be making bad food choices.

3 It's a great way to break up the stresses of the morning and afternoon workday. It's an investment in the productivity of your afternoon.

Lunchtime workouts are constrained by time and the facilities you have available. For these reasons, our lunchtime workout is for a total of just 30 minutes and can be performed either outdoors or inside a health club.

Have your gear ready and try to plan your morning to minimise the possibility of last-minute problems preventing you from training. Don't eat in the hour preceding your workout. If possible be moving around during this period rather than glued to your desk and keep as warm as you can so that you will at least have achieved a passive warm up. An extra layer of clothing will help achieve this.

Divide your time as follows:

Minute	Activity
0–5	warm up
6–15	aerobic training (entrée)
16–25	muscular conditioning (main course)
26–30	warm down and relaxation (dessert)

The clocks hit noon and off you go. If you've changed into your gear in the office, your workout starts now. Take the stairs instead of the lift and out into the fresh air as soon as you can. Jog for 2 minutes to increase blood flow and elevate muscle temperature. It's a minimum, though this still will be sufficient to initiate a sweating response and faster respiration.

Stop and stretch against a convenient wall for 3 minutes. If you hold your stretches for 8 seconds and quickly change from one exercise to the next when the 8 seconds is up, you will have time for 18 stretches. Once again, it's a minimum, but it will prepare you for the aerobic work to come.

If you've walked to a health club and changed there before starting your workout, the same principles apply, though you would use a bike or preferably a treadmill to warm up. Rowing and stepping are best left until after you have stretched. By the way, the image of health clubs has changed a lot over the past few years. You no longer have to get fit before you can walk into a gym. You can now actually go there to get fit!

If you're training for the full 30 minutes outdoors, walking or running are the obvious choices, though in some public areas there are bikes, rowers and arm grinders provided for public usage. If you're walking, keep your tempo at the desired rate of 1 kilometre each 7 or 8 minutes. Rowing on a river or swimming in a pool are both possibilities, but they take precious time to get organised and active.

If you are running, try this 'run through' drill. Set yourself the task of 10 run throughs, starting 'on the minute'. This is most easily organised if you estimate a 'track' of approximately 80 metres. The concept of the session is to stride the distance along your track and then recover before striding back the other way at the start of the next minute. The faster you do your stride, the more time you have to rest before the minute is up and you have to run back the other way. If you need more of a challenge, make the strides a slightly longer distance. If it's too tough, drop the distance back to 60 metres.

If you're capable of an even more demanding workout, try to complete each of your strides in between 15 to 18 seconds. Then jog back to your starting point in the remaining 45 to 48 seconds, before starting the next stride 'on the minute'.

In the first drill you run one way, rest and then run back the other way at the start of the next minute. In the second variation you run one way and jog back all within a minute, and then keep repeating the up and back exercise as each new minute ticks over. You cover twice as much distance the second way so make sure you are up to it before you try it.

If you're back in the gym, use your favourite electronic equipment to achieve the same effect. Accelerate for 20 second 'spurts,' then return to steady pacing for the next 40 seconds of each minute. This type of interval training works well when time is of the essence.

You are now half-way through your workout. The next 10 minutes are devoted to keeping some tone and shape in your muscles. This is the 'muscles for main'. The following routine applies either in the gym or on a park bench.

Time	Exercise	Description
0–30 secs	Step ups	Step one foot onto the bench then drive the other forcefully upward in a jumping type motion. Alternate lead leg each time.
0.5–1 min	Dips	Hands on the bench, feet outstretched so you are in a semi-sitting position. Lower buttocks to ground and return. Repeat.
1–1.5 min	Squats	Hold onto bench for balance. Bend knees into squat while back is kept as straight as possible. Pause for one second at deepest point of squat. Raise and repeat.
1.5–2 min	Push ups	Either with knees on ground or with hands on bench to elevate the upper body.
2–3 min	Abdominals	Raise your feet onto the bench. Cross hands on chest and lift upper body toward knees. Pause for one second at top, lower and repeat.
3–4 min	Calf raises	Hold bench for balance, with one foot off the ground. Raise fully up onto the toes of the working foot, pause for one second, lower and repeat. Change legs after 30 seconds.
4–4.5 min	Twisting push ups	Start on your back in a half reclining position. Turn your body to the left, take your weight with your hands and push back up into a sitting position. Repeat on other side.

4.5–5 min	Twisting sit ups	Feet elevated on bench. Hands crossed on chest. Raise and turn upper body to the left, hold for one second, lower and repeat to other side. Works oblique abdominals.
5–5.5 min	Step ups	Step one foot onto the bench then drive the other forcefully upward in a jumping type motion. Alternate lead leg each time.
5.5–6 min	Dips	Hands on the bench, feet outstretched so you are in a semi-sitting position. Lower buttocks to ground and return. Repeat.
6–6.5 min	Squats	Hold onto bench for balance. Bend knees into squat while back is kept as straight as possible. Pause for one second at deepest point of squat. Raise and repeat.
6.5–7 min	Push ups	Either with knees on ground or with hands on bench to elevate upper body.
7–8 min	Abdominals	Raise your feet onto the bench. Cross hands on chest and lift upper body toward knees. Pause for one second at top, lower and repeat.
8–9 min	Calf raises	Hold bench for balance, with one foot off the ground. Raise fully up onto the toes of the working foot, pause for one second, lower and repeat. Change legs after 30 seconds.
9–9.5 min	Twisting push ups	Start on your back in a half reclining position. Turn your body to the left, take your weight with your hands and push back up into a sitting position. Repeat on other side.
9.5–10 min	Twisting sit ups	Feet elevated on bench. Hands crossed on chest. Raise and turn upper body to the left, hold for one second, lower and repeat to other side.

Please remember that all the exercises are done for time rather than repetitions. As long as you keep moving you will be earning exercise points. Keep a visible clock handy or lay your watch down in front of you to keep track of the time. Move immediately from one exercise and set up for the next exercise without a break.

There are 5 minutes to go in your lunchtime workout. Use this time to slowly walk around and control your pulse rate by breathing evenly and deeply. Include a few gentle stretches and try to release tension as you stretch. This is your de-stressing dessert. After 3 minutes, find a place where you can lie or sit quietly and just enjoy having earned 2 more exercise points.

Congratulate yourself on the workout you've just completed. If you can manage it, keep your focus away from the dramas that await you back 'in real life'. The office can wait for a minute or two. You've just done something good and you deserve to enjoy it. My motto has always been: 'If you can't have free time, at least have me time!'

Please make sure you take in some good food some time during the morning or early in the afternoon. Don't skip lunch altogether.

THE GREAT SIX

Here are six basic ideas to help implement some practical day-to-day activity in your life.

1 Earn your breakfast. Do something physical when you first wake and before you eat. This will burn kilojoules while also suppressing your appetite. If a 15-minute walk or jog (1 point) doesn't appeal to you, try 10 sets of the following: 10 push ups, 10 sit ups, 10 back rolls, 10 knee twists and 10 toe touches (15 minutes = 1 point).

2 Move every 2 hours. If you have a sedentary job, make sure you stimulate your metabolism at least every 2 hours with a walk around the office or down the stairs. It only takes a minute to elevate your metabolism but the results are much longer lasting.

3 At lunchtime, don't just eat. Your aim is to keep your metabolism working so that you'll be burning energy even when you're resting. At least walk somewhere to buy or eat your lunch, even if this means walking around the block before eating in the lunchroom next door to your office.

4 Never allow yourself more than 48 hours of inactivity. Make this a hard and fast rule. If it's been 2 days since you've trained, then it's time to train now, even if it's 10 o'clock at night or 6 o'clock in the morning.

5 Try this activity either as a walking or running session on a 100-metre course marked at 20-metre intervals.

Start at one end, and then follow this pattern: Fast for 20 metres, slow for 80 metres.

You can either walk or run to this pattern as long as you alter your speed between fast and slow tempos.

Turn around and start in the opposite direction.
Fast for 40 metres, slow for 60 metres.
Turn around and start in the opposite direction.
Fast for 60 metres, slow for 40 metres.
Turn around and start in the opposite direction.
Fast for 80 metres, slow for 20 metres.
Turn around and start in the opposite direction.
Fast for 100 metres.
Turn around and start in the opposite direction.
Slow for 100 metres.

Turn around and start again from the beginning. One circuit will take you 6 minutes if walking and approximately 4 minutes if you are running. See how many circuits you can complete in 30 minutes. This will earn you 2 exercise points. Sandwich this between a 15-minute walk at the start and a 15-minute walk at the end for a workout total of 60 minutes and 4 points.

6   Try this as a strength-training program. Every time you stop at traffic lights, do an isometric strength exercise. Alternate between pushing the steering wheel in from the outsides, pulling out from the insides, pulling up and downward by holding the top and bottom of the wheel, and squeezing one part of the steering wheel between both hands. Do the first exercise at the first set of lights, the second exercise at the next set of lights, and so on.

Keep alternating whenever you're forced to stop at lights. Remember that every contraction counts. You won't score exercise points unless the lights break down and leave you stuck on red for 15 minutes, though it will keep exercise at the forefront of your consciousness.

ODDBALL WORKOUTS

Sometimes you'll feel like sitting instead of sweating, and the thought of doing something like walking 5 kilometres will leave you uninspired. Do not despair. When this happens to you, it will be time to try something different to earn your exercise points. It's a very positive thing to use some variety while still counting exercise points. The oddball workouts will achieve a training effect. They will increase your heart rate continuously for 15 minutes.

They are simple, safe and effective and they are all worth 1 exercise point for every 15 minutes you spend on them.

GOLF

This is not what you are thinking. Grab your nine iron and a ball and head for the practice fairway (walk if it's close enough). The idea is to chip and run the ball 20 metres each time you strike it. Walk briskly to the ball, quickly line it up and again chip it as close to 20 metres as you can. It should take you 10 shots to reach the 200 metre marker on the practice fairway. Turn around and try to return to your starting point in exactly 10 more shots.

Try it again, chipping 40 or 50 metres each time. You should complete 4 or 5 circuits (up to the 200 metre mark and back) in 15 minutes. You will have covered 2 kilometres in good time and it might even improve your game! I often call this the 'put on, take off' workout because you increase your exercise scores while decreasing your golf scores.

ANY CHILDREN?

Grab a child, preferably your own, and a ball (the smaller the child the bigger the ball) and walk to the nearest park. Stand 2 metres apart and toss the ball to and fro. You'll probably end up doing quite a bit of chasing and retrieving from misdirected throws but it's great fun.

If the child is a hot shot thrower, have him or her aim the ball a metre or so to your left or right so that you'll have to move to take the pass. Quickly steady, then return the throw, but not so fast that the child doesn't see it coming. How many catches can you take before the ball is dropped? Fifteen minutes of this activity will provide a training effect and improve your reflexes, and it's fun. The simplest things sometimes really are the best.

Whenever you can turn play into points, you are ahead of the game.

THE OUT AND BACK HIKE

Sorry folks, it does involve walking or jogging; however, it is different. You can also do this: swimming, cycling, roller blading, scootering or pogo hopping.

The out and back hike involves travelling as far as you can in 8 minutes. When the 8 minutes has elapsed make a mental note of where you are (your outmark), then turn around and head back to the start. You have to try to make it back to the start within the next 8 minutes.

The next time you make the hike on the same route, you have to try to beat your out-mark and then still make it back to the start in the following 8 minutes. The short-term goal of always trying to reach your out-mark and then still return home in the prescribed time provides great motivation. Give it a try. It's tough work and it will really keep you honest.

DO I HEAR SOMETHING RIPPING?

This 'loosely arranged' flexibility and movement circuit is ideal for an indoor session when you need a change. There is no escape, even if it's too cold and wet for you outside!

When you perform a stretching session adopt a smooth and rhythmic manner and avoid bouncing or jerking. Make sure you aren't invading other people's personal space when you start to stretch. There is a chance that there will be some strange noises and gases escaping from all over the place. Don't be embarrassed — this is a natural thing; just turn the radio up and leave a window open.

Keep moving and don't be afraid to throw in some push ups and a few sit ups as well. Try toe touches, knee bends, side bends and whatever else you recall from your school phys. ed. days. Stretching should be informal and relaxed so don't follow a strictly preset routine; just stretch whatever feels tight.

A couple of things to remember: never hold your breath, and whenever you're on your back keep your knees bent to protect your back. Go to it.

REBOUNDS

If you can get hold of a tennis ball or similar, and have access to a brick wall or retaining wall, then you have what it takes for rebounds. Serious athletes use this very activity to develop hand-eye co-ordination and reflexes. For the time being we'll just worry about trying to catch the ball.

Stand 3 metres from the wall. Bend your knees so you are ready to react quickly and pitch the ball underarm at the wall. With any luck it will rebound in your general direction. Try to catch it! If you do, throw it again immediately. If that's too easy, throw harder, or catch one-handed or clap twice before the ball returns. Whatever you do, keep challenging yourself so that you keep moving. You'll spend a fair amount of time chasing the ball from uneven bounces and dropped catches. Make sure you jog (or walk briskly) after the ball and then back to position. Doesn't sound too strenuous? You might be surprised.

You can try the same activity with a tennis racquet and ball.

FART WHO? FARTLEK!

Fartlek means 'speed play' and was invented in Sweden a few decades ago. It's a type of conditioning which involves changing pace while you're moving. For example, if you are walking along the street you might jog for two street signs distance, walk for one street sign and then jog again for the next two. You continue with this pattern for 15 minutes to an hour to score 1–4 exercise points respectively.

As you progress you could jog for 2 street signs, stride to the next, jog for the next 2, then have a walk recovery for 1 street sign. Design the walk/jog/stride combination to suit your current fitness level. Start conservatively and gradually build up.

It's a great shame to see people grimacing and 'over-focused' when walking or jogging. Don't push yourself past mild discomfort. The intensity should be no greater than 7 out of 10 on your scale of perceived exertion (or 70% of your maximum heart rate if you have a monitor). The demands of your workout should not be severe enough to be obvious to an onlooker. Over the years, at least 100 people must have told me that they won't start running until they finally see their first happy jogger. You could be the one! You have to try to enjoy it rather than endure it. You may even convert a few others.

The physical benefits of walking and jogging are matched by therapeutic factors. These include reductions in blood pressure, muscle tension, skin temperature and the flushing of metabolic wastes from the muscles, liver and bloodstream. You will inhibit this natural stress release if you are over-exerted or tense. Don't fight it. Help your body to release tension.

Finally, please don't walk or run along busy roads during times of peak hour traffic! Apart from the potential hazard of being skittled by an overloaded bus, it's unhealthy. You will be breathing the concentrated ingredients of city smog, gases that are also favoured substances for committing suicide. A 30-minute exposure to this environment of hydrogen cyanide and carbon monoxide while inhaling 20 times or more each minute is like chain-smoking a pack of unfiltered cigarettes. You won't be instilling oxygen into your lungs, bloodstream and muscles; you will be injecting poison. If you don't have another option, don't train. This is one of the very rare cases where inactivity is preferable to activity. If you can, find a park and a soft surface. We want you to carry on, not become carrion!

ANYONE FOR TENNIS?

A star you mightn't be but after 15 minutes of this activity you'll be ready for anything. The idea's simple. You play in the normal manner (serving underarm if you have trouble in this area), but you jog to retrieve the ball after each rally. This may not seem like much of a change but for the average tennis player it more than doubles the active component of the game. Fifteen minutes may be more than ample when you start, so keep an eye on your watch as well as the ball. Don't try for a full '4-point hour' if you're not ready for it.

Please work at an appropriate rate in any of the oddball workouts you use. As a rule of thumb, when you are exercising you should still be able to carry on a conversation but not without some pauses for breathing. If you can talk without interruption you are probably not working hard enough and if you can't talk at all then you are definitely working too hard.

As an example, when you are kite flying, don't sprint 60 metres into the wind then stand admiring the sky for 5 minutes. Take your time, walk briskly and keep moving. When the kite falls, retrieve it quickly and start over. Keep an eye on your watch and continue the procedure for 15 minutes. All of these are aerobic activities (sorry, that's jargon), which really just means that you are working at a steady and continuous level that is within your body's oxygen usage capabilities.

When you go beyond the point known as anaerobic threshold (more jargon), you enter the realm where you actually use up more oxygen than you can take in. This is called anaerobic activity (without oxygen) and you can only work anaerobically for one minute or so before you have to slow down and pay back the debt of oxygen you have built up.

Kite flying is just an example. If you have the dog out in the park, don't tease him into a frenzy until you have to climb a tree for safety or lie down for a rest. Toss him a ball or take him on a lead and remember to keep moving at a rate you will be able to sustain for at least the magic 15 minutes. Whether it's a crawl, walk, jog, stride or sprint depends on you. You'll be surprised how quickly you will progress.

All activity will still be beneficial, especially if you enjoy it. For every 15-minute segment when you have more activity time than rest time, you will score 1 exercise point. If you can string together 4 of these 15-minute time segments into an hour of exercise you will score 4 exercise points. When you manage to do this 4 times each week in combination with 12 daily food points, you'll be two thirds of the way along your journey to the Health Zone.

What do I do now?

1 Be aware of the fat content, in grams, of the food you eat during the course of the day. Keep using the food tables in Appendix 2 to help your knowledge. Practise counting food points each day.

2 Think about your exercise in terms of 1 point for every 15 minutes spent when you are active more than you are resting.

3 Use what's left of the 2-week transition period to build up your exercise points to 4 points per day on 4 days each week.

4 Aim for one day in the next week when you score 12 food points and 4 exercise points on the same day.

5 Congratulate yourself if you achieve this worthwhile feat! You are two thirds of the way to the Health Zone already.

7

THE HIDDEN AGING AGENT

*'A fanatic is someone who won't change his or her
mind and can't change the subject.'*

WINSTON CHURCHILL

FINDING A MIRROR THAT WORKS

The greatest challenge in using Every Day Counts is being
honest with yourself. It can be tough to give yourself
straight answers to questions such as: 'Did I actually train
long enough to earn my 4 exercise points for today?'
'Have I really made enough good nutrition choices to
score my 12 food points?' and 'How much work time do I
spend thinking about home and how much home time do
I spend thinking or worrying about work?'

Perhaps the hardest question of all to answer is, 'Am I
able to relax and control my stress levels?' I must have
asked people that question over 1000 times, and out of all
those people only four have openly admitted to me that
they don't cope well with stress. That's one person in
every 250 admitting that stress is an issue in their lives.

People have been telling me for years that they sleep
like a baby! Finally I worked out what they meant: they

sleep for an hour, wake up and cry for an hour, sleep for an hour, and so on, just like a baby.

People tell me that they live a balanced lifestyle. I recently met a financial advisor who told me that he'd gone for the 'lifestyle option' in his new job. 'I'm home by 8 most nights, I only work until 2 on Saturdays and I have every second Sunday off,' he told me proudly.

I'd hate to have seen the hours he worked in his previous job!

Figure A illustrates my idea of Utopia. It's when we balance our career or home responsibilities with time for personal development and time for our support systems.

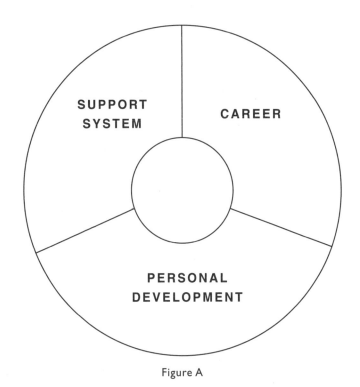

Figure A

Career is important. It enables us to feel that we are contributing to society in a manner that fosters our self-esteem. It also helps us provide for ourselves and our loved ones. This is why a career as a parent at home is tough. There is very little recognition, either friendly or otherwise.

The Personal Development sphere of life means spending time with your friends, pursuing your hobbies, learning new skills, giving back to the community and generally gathering wisdom as you go through your life.

The Support System sphere is our health: the very thing that allows us to be successful and an achiever in the other areas of our life.

Without time for our personal development and support systems, we become one-dimensional and imbalanced.

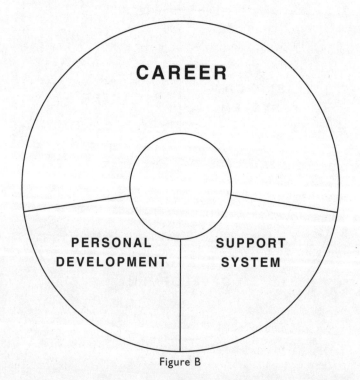

Figure B

Many people who see themselves as being balanced appear to me to be spending so much time and effort on their career, parents included, that there is simply not enough left for personal development and the support system. What I see is Figure B.

There are only 24 hours in a day. Time management and sleep deprivation can only go so far. Sometimes the people closest to the fire are the last ones to feel the heat. If Figure B describes your life, you are under attack from stress.

Newsflash: Stress is an issue in all our lives.

Feel the nape of your neck with the palm of your hand! How warm does it feel? One of the direct physical effects of anxiety is a decrease in blood flow to peripheral areas such as your fingertips, nose and ears, and the skin at the back of your neck. This causes a decrease in the temperature of your skin, which will be noticeably cooler to your touch. If the area between your shoulder blades feels cooler than your chest, shoulders or back, then you could be in a state of stress! The old saying 'hot under the collar' would be more accurate if it were 'cold under the collar'! Try this simple 'neck test' next time your schedule gets overcrowded, your budget tight or there is some tension at home. If you feel this area with your hand and it is noticeably cooler, it's an indication that you are having a stress attack!

We will never eliminate pressure from our lives, and we wouldn't want to even if we could. This chapter is dedicated to controlling *pressure* so that it doesn't turn into *stress*.

I've already told a number of stories about other people in the previous chapters. Well, here's a story about myself. I don't handle pressure well. I admit it. I turn problems over and over in my mind and when I allow myself to become over-anxious it effects my mood, sleep, appetite and entire outlook on life. I used to think of this state as being nervous rather than being stressed. As a junior sportsman I would look forward to my football or cricket games all week only to wake up feeling tired, slow and heavy on the morning of the game. I would be so determined to do well that when the game or exam finally came around, I would be too worked up to perform. I had literally played myself out before the real action started.

I've carried these same traits into adulthood. As a young man I would allow myself to get keyed up over things and at times I would become over-awed by fear of failure. I had a short career in the then VFL, now the AFL. Playing games in front of big crowds for me wasn't just exciting, it was intimidating. Even now I still get nervous before an important meeting or a corporate presentation. Today a casual game of golf can still cause my stomach butterflies to flutter when the gamesmanship starts: that is, if I let it!

Like someone who suffers from migraines or epilepsy, my challenge is to recognise the early warning signs so that I stay in control. I know what I have to do. Counting food and exercise points comes naturally to me; I enjoy it and don't find the discipline overly demanding. However, when I was first developing and experimenting with the Every Day Counts program, I really had to work hard to make myself take the time to score pressure points. I call them pressure points because they deal with *pressure* and prevent *stress*. Now that I have established the habit, I try to block pressure from ever becoming stress. I take the time for a massage, deep breathing session, spa or meditation. These things are now as natural to me as going for a run, lifting some weights or choosing an apple over an éclair.

Even so, there are situations I still find potentially stressful. Heavy traffic is one. I hate being in an environment where there is much frustration, inactivity and latent aggression. The antagonistic and aggressive looks on people's faces infect me with frustration. I feel the pressure. It's an exception when someone gives up just 2 seconds to allow someone else to change lanes or enter the traffic flow. I think that we see society at its worst on our roads.

Things like this can really get to me . . . if I let them. It's my choice. Those traits are there in my personality, but I choose how I react to the things that threaten to stimulate these stress responses.

The stimulus for stress is still there. It's called pressure. The response is my choice! It only becomes stress when I allow it to be.

Most people deny stress rather then deal with stress. What I see as an observer of people under stress is not the same as they see themselves. You have to find a mirror that works. You have to be honest with yourself.

STRESS AND YOU

It's said that alcoholics and compulsive gamblers can't begin their rehabilitation until they admit there is a problem. Well, I have a stress problem. I also try to deal with it by taking 20 minutes to score 4 pressure points every day.

Even life-long habits can be changed. If you are a natural worrier, try to reduce your worrying by 50% each year. You can divide something in half every year forever and it will never disappear, it will always be there, but only as a tiny fraction of what it used to be. Worry is like that. You may never eliminate it from your personality, but it will be well and truly under control.

Let's find out if you have the type of personality that leaves you vulnerable to converting pressure to stress. Please give yourself an honest *yes* or *no* answer to each of these 10 questions.

1 Do you prefer the driver's seat to
   the passenger's seat?   Yes/No
   (because you are in control)
2 Do you intensely dislike being late?   Yes/No
   (because it's a weakness)
3 Do you tend to internalise emotions?   Yes/No
   (it's a sign of weakness or an inability to cope if you
   show emotion)
4 Do you have trouble delegating?   Yes/No
   (no one will do it as well as you — and it's quicker
   to do it yourself)
5 Do you see the task ahead rather
   than the work achieved?   Yes/No
   (like the mountaineer with an unquenchable desire
   for the next challenge)
6 Do you react well to time and deadline
   pressure?   Yes/No
   (if you want something done, ask a busy person)
7 Do you take the side streets just to keep
   moving?   Yes/No
   (you drive an extra few kilometres, you use more
   petrol and you take more time, but at least you
   don't have to stop at those damn traffic lights)
8 Do you work better alone?   Yes/No
   (others distract you and dilute your workload)
9 Do you love lists?   Yes/No
   (it's a measure of achievement throughout the day)

10 Do you really love lists?   Yes/No
(You must answer yes to this final question if you've ever been working from a list and you suddenly remember something you've already done, but it wasn't included on your list. You then write it down, just so you get the chance to cross it off!)

If you have answered *yes* to five or more of these questions, then, like me, it's no longer a matter of whether or not you are confronted by the stress that pressure can bring — you are! It's now a matter of what you are going to do about it. If you answered *yes* to three or four questions there are still some benefits to be gained by using techniques to counter pressure and prevent stress in your life.

If you answered *yes* to only one or two questions, you are pretty laid back. In fact you're so laid back you wouldn't care what your score was anyway! You may not see what all the fuss is about because stress stimuli don't create a stress response in you. Congratulations!

COUNTING PRESSURE POINTS

The third step to living in the Health Zone and making Every Day Count is to spend 20 minutes of quiet, relaxation or renewal time every day to control pressure in your life. You score 1 pressure point for every 5 minutes you spend on any 'anxiety abating activity'. I'll give you some examples shortly.

The conscious mind is constantly striving to achieve more and more. The subconscious mind is trying to tell us to slow our respiratory and heart rates, reduce our blood pressure and relax muscle tension. It's the id and the ego. By taking some regular quiet time, we allow the messages from our subconscious mind to enter the conscious mind and allow these positive physical changes to take place. That's why taking time to deal with pressure works so effectively.

Up until now we have considered our physical being only from an eating and an exercise viewpoint. It's natural for us to have a desire to protect our health, to look good, feel good, perform well and hold off the aging process. To do this we cannot ignore the non-physical, because the ways we think have enormous influences on the way we are. Stress and worry can be the most insidious aging agents of all.

It's not just what you're eating, it's what's eating you. It's not just that you exercise, it's how you exercise your mind. To counter the physical results of stress, we need the ability to choose our own thoughts. We must develop the skills to ensure that the pressure of a stress stimulus doesn't always create a stress response.

Stress isn't the beginning of the chain, it's the end of the chain. Stress is a physical response to what too often is an emotional stimulus. When a cat jumps in front of your car or you are physically threatened in some way, you want to have a stress response. The stress response is a release of adrenaline from the adrenal gland and free floating fatty acids from the liver.

It happens in a fraction of a second, but it gives us speed, power and decisiveness. If you could bottle these secretions they would be the greatest performance enhancers of all time.

Incredible things can be achieved when we have a stress response. A small woman in London lifted the rear of car weighing half a tonne to free a trapped baby. An old man ran 5 kilometres in less than 20 minutes to raise the alarm when his wife was hurt in a car accident on a country road. These are actual documented cases of superhuman performances induced by stress.

In my own youth a sun-baking snake startled a friend and myself. We vaulted over a 1.5-metre fence in a split second to get away. We cleared that fence by so far you would have thought we had a pole vault and a 30-metre run up. We were over it before we knew it. There wasn't a moment's thought or a moment's hesitation. The snake was definitely a Type B personality: it couldn't have cared less. All the panic and stress was on the human side! I'm sure you have your own experiences of 'action under fire'.

In an environment where we can respond in a physical manner, stress can be a very positive thing! That's why many people play sport. We seek the stress, the outlet and the action! Sometimes we just have to let it out. The saying 'burning off some steam' is really quite accurate.

Now think of a time when you've heard a sudden noise during the night or you've narrowly missed being in a traffic accident. The danger, if there ever was any, has passed and you are left feeling jumpy and unsettled. It takes a long time to settle down after an experience like that. You sit in your car shaking or you lie awake in bed for hours. You are literally stewing in your own juices.

The physical responses to a stress stimulus are not healthy in the sedentary environment of the office or the home. It's not just an emotional feeling; it's a physical reaction. What do you think happens to the adrenaline and the fatty acids if we can't respond physically when we do have a stress episode? Unfortunately for us, these secretions only gradually dissipate from the bloodstream. It's like stirring up the fine particles in a glass of water. Hold the glass up to the light and watch these particles slowly sink back to the bottom of the glass. Stress sinks to our blood vessel walls, and it stays there!

In the short term these effects can include a feeling of agitation and jumpiness, tight muscles, especially in the shoulders, shallow rapid breathing and elevated pulse. In the long term the results can be far more serious: high blood pressure, elevated blood fats, skin irritations and rashes, hunched posture and more. It is a most unhealthy scenario for someone working in a sedentary environment to be eliciting a stress response on a daily basis if there is no opportunity for the stress secretions to be utilised.

Remember ... don't get angry. *Anger* is only one letter away from *danger*.

STRESS AND THE HEALTH ZONE

Living in the Health Zone is a holistic concept. We are a package. We cannot separate the physical from the emotional or the spiritual. Healthy body may promote healthy mind, but it won't if you're so worried about keeping to a schedule or making it to that extra workout that you eat up your insides with anxiety.

You won't find the Health Zone or score enough points to keep with the program if you spend a disproportionate amount of time on the physical when compared to what you spend on meditation, relaxation, prayer, massage, spa, tai chi or daydreaming. You must give your subconscious mind time to get involved in your being. Your requirement is 4 points per day and each point takes up to 5 minutes to earn.

It's the subconscious mind that is telling us to relax, dilate our blood vessels, to reduce blood pressure, slow and deepen our breathing and reduce the tension in our toes, fingers, shoulders and jaw.

It's the conscious mind that's always telling us to make deadlines, climb the ladder and achieve more success. There's nothing wrong with being an achiever, in sport, fitness, business and life, but you have to pace yourself.

There is no point climbing to the top of the tree if there is no view from up there. Make sure the ladder of success is leaning against the right wall before you start the climb.

Try to catch yourself at an unsuspecting moment. Freeze. Are your jaws or teeth tightly clenched, is your brow furrowed and are your hands balled into fists? If it's a *yes* to any of these, it's an indicator that you're not as relaxed as you may think you are.

Please set yourself the challenge of totally clearing your mind for 30 seconds. Try it when you get to the end of this paragraph. This basic test requires you to prevent any one particular thought from staying in your consciousness. As soon as a thought about, say, your car being due for a service, or a report you have to prepare gains your attention, you must push it out of your consciousness and clear your mind. Thoughts will come and go, though you must aim to keep specific things from returning and disturbing your respite. Your aim is not to think about anything. See if you can get someone to do the timing for you. Your 30 seconds starts now!

How did you go? It's not as easy as it would seem, is it? So no one's perfect. If you have already learned how to meditate you may have been successful in clearing your mind for 30 seconds. However, you certainly aren't in the minority if you discovered tension in your body and you had difficulty keeping your mind clear.

Don't be fooled into thinking that stress is an emotional condition. It's actually a physical response to what too often is an emotional stimulus.

Sometimes we need to respond to pressure. This is when stress is positive. We want to react to a physical stress stimulus like a bus coming through a stop sign. It's then that we need our entire physical being to be on full alert so we can respond quickly and strongly enough to protect ourselves. It works the same way in sport and in business when we want to be at our best. The old saying, 'fire in the belly,' is very, very apt.

What we don't want is to be in this state of full arousal when there is no opportunity for release of the products of stress, the adrenaline and free floating fatty acids. These secretions can only be dissipated or used up through a physical outlet. That fire in the belly has to burn something and we don't want it to be the lining of our stomach.

When we feel stressed, what we're really experiencing is a tensing and tightening of our muscles, an increase in blood flow to the core of the body, a heightening of nerve impulses, an increase in blood pressure and a quickening and shallowing effect on our breathing. In short, we're ready for a fight, and if we allow ourselves to remain in this state of anxiety for too long, sooner or later we're likely to go looking for one!

Being on edge like this is a lot less healthy than having an occasional chocolate bar or a gin and tonic with dinner! To successfully make Every Day Count you must integrate sensible eating and exercise with techniques and time to recognise and control anxiety.

Some people actually create stress for themselves by trying so hard to eat the right things that they worry, fret and feel guilty when they eat the slightest nutritional impurity. There is a point where the worry becomes more physically damaging than the poor food choice itself. It's the *illusion* end of the lifestyle pendulum.

Remember, it's not just what you're eating, it's what's eating you!

What do I do now?

We can change our focus away from tension and anxiety back to a more neutral state. We don't have to be as relaxed as a meditating yogi is, though we should be able to control our emotional state at least 90% of the time. This is your challenge. It also makes the third aspect of Every Day Counts, scoring pressure points, vital.

For the other 10%, when things really start to get to you, the productive thing is to recognise that you are stressed and concentrate on burning up the stress secretions through a physical outlet. Don't hold back the torrent or try to deny the physical state you are in.

In the next chapter, you'll learn techniques to deal with pressure and techniques to deal with stress.

Don't stew in your own juices. Don't burn in your own fire. Prevention is better than cure, yes, though there will still be times when it gets to you.

Let it out!

8

PRESSURE POINTS AND STRESS SCORES

'I was seldom able to see an opportunity until it had ceased to become one.'

MARK TWAIN

ANXIETY ABATERS

We know that pressure is always going to be a factor in our lives. We also know that we can stop this pressure from degenerating into stress. Now let's turn our attention to exactly what we can do to keep control of pressure and stress and earn those all important 4 pressure points each day. The many techniques available to you can be classified as:

- preventing a stress response, or
- reacting to a stress response.

PREVENTING A STRESS RESPONSE

Let's concentrate first on preventing pressure from turning into stress. There are 4 anxiety abaters for you to try when this is your aim. These techniques are useful in preventing pressure (a stimulus for stress) that is already present from creating a physical stress reaction inside your body. These are immediate minute-by-minute techniques to incorporate into your day. Each is worth 1 point every time it is used, even if you don't need the full 5 minutes. These techniques pay immediate dividends.

I like to think of a stress stimulus having to get past my defences before it succeeds in creating a stress response. These defences are like an outer ring that I use to protect myself. A stress response only occurs when this outer rim is pierced. I have 4 stress defenders. Here they are.

RECOGNITION

My first stress defence is simply to be aware of a stress stimulus when it rears its ugly head. If I don't know how to recognise the enemy, how am I going to protect myself? My stress blockers can't work if I don't call them into action. If I only recognise stress when it is a response rather than a stimulus, my reaction is no longer a matter of defence; it's a matter of damage control.

Recognising the stimuli for stress in your life is as simple as writing a list. For me the list includes heavy traffic and insufficient preparation time before I give a presentation. For some people it's the mindless chatter of breakfast disc jockeys or out of control children at dinnertime. For you it might be too many meetings, no 'me time' or the antics of people you come into contact with. You know yourself well enough to identify the things that are likely to cause you aggravation.

Your first line of defence is to see these stimuli for what they are. They are sources of pressure and they have the potential to produce a stress response, though you don't have to always let it happen. There is nothing in the world more common than unfulfilled potential so why not let the potential for stress go unfulfilled? Just by recognising your stress precursors, you will go a long way toward defusing them. Keep your guard up.

When you find yourself under pressure, recognise it and let it go. If you are caught at a red light, you can get as mad as you like, but the red light doesn't care. When someone at work is frustrating you, recognise it and let it go. Don't get stressed unless it's going to help.

Stress defender number 1: Recognition

LAUGH LINES

My next defence against the things that cause stress is to laugh at them. Laughing is a physical release and a muscle relaxant. Be like Batman or James Bond: they laugh in the face of danger. We must learn to laugh in the stead of anger. It's a great technique because it's directly under our control; we don't need any equipment or preparation and it takes no longer to laugh than it does to frown or curse.

Laughing is a stress-stopping technique used by many successful people. If you have a computer breakdown in your office or your car starts making a funny noise the day you are due to go on a driving holiday, your reaction can't fix the problem by itself. You can get angry and frustrated if you want to, but you'll still have to call the technician or the mechanic. Choose your own thoughts. We have to look closely for the humour and irony in our daily lives.

Laughing or smiling when I'm confronted by something unpleasant and out of my direct control is my second line of defence. It will feel weird and unnatural when you first try it and if you happen to be near a mirror your laughter will appear false and forced. That's because it is. Please persevere; this technique works like a charm.

You'll still need the mechanic to repair your car but you'll be protecting yourself against your own breakdown.

The laughter must last for at least five seconds. It's not enough to force a smile and quick 'ha-ha'. The minimum is 10 'ha's'. That's 'ha-ha-ha-ha-ha-ha-ha-ha-ha-ha'. You won't feel like doing it when the pressure mounts, but it's exactly what you must do. Think of something funny or just start laughing. All you have to lose is a stress attack.

Stress defender number 2: Laughter

YOUR CIRCLE OF INFLUENCE

The third defence mechanism is a thought process known as operating in your 'circle of influence'. Consider how we think. Also consider this: some things we can control directly by our actions, others we can't. When you are thinking about what you are going to have for breakfast, which route you are going to take in your car and what you are going to watch tonight on television, you are thinking and operating in your circle of influence. You can directly control these things, that is if the kids don't hide the remote control. You have the power to take action and choose between the alternatives before you.

When you are thinking about the boss's office decor or famine in developing countries you are thinking within what is known as your 'circle of concern'. Your circle of concern includes the thousands of things we often think about but have no direct control over. When threatened by a stimulus for stress, it is unproductive to operate in our circle of concern. Of course this does not mean that we should never think about these things. As humans we are thinking beings. However, as our third line of defence is designed to prevent a stress stimulus from becoming a stress response, when recognition and laughter don't work, we should force ourselves to think only about the things we have some control over.

I recently spoke to a group of former executives who had resigned or been made redundant. As part of the career transition program they were involved in, many reported that they found unsuccessful job interviews to be very stressful experiences. They mused and mulled over why they hadn't been hired and they felt that they must have done something wrong in the way they presented either their resumes or themselves. They were allowing a genuine stimulus for stress to become a stress response. They were thinking and operating in their circles of concern. They were stewing in their own juices. Of course they would have liked to win the position, but once the decision went against them, there was nothing to be gained by getting anxious or angry about it.

I urged them to focus on their circles of influence. What could they control? What positive action could they take? They could ask for feedback from the prospective employer. They could make a genuine inquiry about their interview performance and why the agency or employer had chosen someone else. They could have their resume reviewed by one of the career transition experts. They could also seek new interview opportunities.

Sometimes you can't directly take action on the issue that's creating the pressure. However, you can take action on something else. As well as being productive for whatever it is you do work on, you'll be occupying your mind and preventing worthless worry.

Feeling helpless is a sure way to convert a stress stimulus into a stress response. Taking action is a sure way to stop yourself from feeling helpless, and thinking in your circle of influence is a short cut to taking action. There is always something you can do.

Easy to say, hard to do? In our lives we all experience mishaps. Some people are unfortunate enough to experience a tragedy. If you experience a real tragedy, you'll know it. Tragedies can't be overcome by thinking within your circle of influence. Tragedies are bigger than that and I would never presume to advise anyone on how to overcome a true tragedy. What I do know is that we can allow ourselves to blow a mishap out of all proportion and turn it into a tragedy in our mind. Operating in your circle of influence can control mishaps. Some people think of it as 'big stuff' and 'little stuff'. A birth, a marriage, a break up in a relationship, a severe illness or a death, they are the big stuff. Maybe a financial crisis is big stuff as well; just maybe it classifies as a tragedy. Everything else is little stuff, things we can either control or we can overcome the effects of.

Most stress stimuli don't even qualify as being mishaps. Things we allowed ourselves to get uptight about last week may not even be remembered today. You have to force yourself to choose your own thoughts. Thinking within your circle of influence is how you choose your thoughts. It's your third line of defence against stress.

Stress defender number 3: Think within your circle of influence

BEST BREATHING

When you sense that your outer rim of protection is letting you down, when your first three defences haven't been effective, it's time to take some deep breaths. This is your fourth and final weapon before the stimulus becomes a stress response.

Breathe in for 3 seconds (a slow count of 1, 2, and 3), hold it for 3 seconds and exhale for 3 seconds. Repeat.

Keep going. Think to yourself 're ...' as you inhale and '...lax' as you exhale. Keep thinking this to yourself as you inhale and exhale. It will take some willpower to make yourself do this for more than a few seconds. Your conscious thoughts will keep trying to regain your concentration, to return your focus to the problem or issue that has created the pressure. Dig in your heels in and stick with the breathing.

Keep your focus on your breathing and your breathing only. Inhale through your nose and exhale through your mouth. Some sportspeople try to focus on inhaling through one nostril and exhaling through the other. The idea is to concentrate on your breathing exclusively until the stimulus for stress recedes. It's impossible to worry while you are focusing hard on each inhalation and exhalation. I find it too difficult to inhale through one nostril and exhale through the other. I concentrate on breathing in through my nose and then out through my mouth.

Controlled breathing sends messages to your subconscious mind to relax your physical channels, to slow your breathing, ease your muscle tension and get your emotional state back to that even, neutral plane we function best in.

The hardest part about controlled breathing is to make yourself do it for long enough. Each 'in for 3, hold for 3 and out for 3' breath cycle tends to last for about 6 seconds because most people count more rapidly than '1 per second'. Ten breath cycles take a minute to complete and you will need at least 2 minutes to break the stress stimulus. This means taking the time to complete 20 breath cycles.

Try it this way. Start the breathing with a mantra type thought like 'in–2–3, hold–2–3, out–2–1'. On the next cycle you say to yourself 'in–2–3, hold–2–3, out–2–2'. On the third cycle you say to yourself 'in–2–3, hold–2–3, out–2–3'. You keep count by the last number you say to yourself on each exhalation. When you get to 'in–2–3, hold–2–3, out–2–20,' you will have made it through the twentieth cycle. Make yourself do it for the full 20 cycles. Take the full 2 minutes.

Stress defender number 4: Best breathing

Now work backwards through your other stress defenders.

Keep your thoughts in your circle of influence. What can you do to take positive action right now? Laugh as you exit that stimulus. Make yourself do the 10 'ha's'. Picture the stimulus moving away from you. This will reinforce the correct mental state and return the control to where it belongs, with you. These anxiety abaters are a great way to block stimuli for stress and they earn you pressure points from within our Every Day Counts system. Your four stress stoppers, in operational order, are:

- to recognise the stimulus
- to laugh at it
- to focus on your circle of influence
- to breathe your way through it.

To score pressure points, our system normally requires you to take 5 minutes of pressure time to earn each point. Sometimes these four weapons won't take that long. The recognition of a stress stimulus being present may only take a few seconds. Even so, with practice this will at times be enough to ensure that the stress stimulus develops no further. You'll stop it dead in its tracks just by seeing it for what it is.

While this may only take you 5 seconds rather than 5 minutes, you have still earned yourself 1 pressure point.

When you block stress like this, you deserve a pressure point. A moment's recognition of stress is worth 5 minutes recuperation. It's a worthwhile exception to our '5 minutes per pressure point' rule. Give yourself the point when you succeed in fighting stress stimuli with your blocking techniques. Keep a mental tally as your day progresses

REACTING TO A STRESS RESPONSE

NEWSFLASH ... incoming!!!! Despite your best efforts, stress is still going to happen. You will develop a resistance to stress, not an immunity. Some stimuli are still going to get through your net. You are still going to get angry and upset, even when it's only a mishap rather than a tragedy.

These are the times when you need an entirely different armoury. It's now too late for your stress blockers. This is when you need 5 minutes to earn each point. This is damage control. This is fightback time.

STRESS AND YOUR SENSES

When the pressure does become stress in your life, think about your 5 senses: sight, hearing, touch, smell and taste. One way to attack stress is to please each of your senses, to act as a pathway to soothe your inner being.

Find something pleasing to look at. Artwork, landscapes, people, architecture, buildings, fish in a tank, even machines work for some people. Select something that's aesthetically pleasing to your eye, and feast on it.

Put on some music that appeals to you. It doesn't have to be soothing sounds from the ocean floor or birds singing in spring; it might be rhythm or even rock. Sounds you enjoy will change your focus away from stress back to stability.

Next, turn your attention to touch. Your tactile sense will revel if it's a whole body experience. Fondling something like a stress ball with your hands is one option. However, your sense of touch will really appreciate larger surface areas of your body being stimulated. Recline in a comfortable chair, lie flat on your back on a carpeted floor or simply self-massage your tension spots. It feels good when it feels good.

Now to the olfactory sense, the sense of smell. Aromatherapy has really opened up the benefits of using our sense of smell to affect our mood. A small amount of oil in a bowl, an oil-scented candle, even a portable facial spray all provide a means to send the right signals to your core.

The final sense is taste. Taste is one sense we naturally pamper in times of stress. The word 'chocoholic' could have been invented for people who seek solace in bonus foods during times of stress. It's a good thing if you recognise the behaviour for what it is and can control it. If you find yourself reaching for the chocolate jar because of stress, have a couple of pieces instead of a couple of dozen, and invest some time in your other senses. It's more effective to pamper yourself with sights, sounds, smell and feel rather than with taste alone. Chocolate is okay, but be aware that each of those tiny cubes can contain 2 grams of fat. When you pamper your taste buds to counter stress, make it a treat and not a tempest: and *EAT SLOWLY*!

STRESS REHAB

I have 5 stress coping techniques to recommend to you when you have succumbed to stress. These are not designed to stop pressure becoming stress; they are designed to help you when you are stressed. All help repair the damage a stress response can cause if you let it go untreated. Remember that the stress response is a physical thing. Everything's up: blood pressure, breathing rate, heart rate, muscle tension and nerve interference. Stress coping combats the physical effects of stress. It cools you down. It gets you back in control after you've lost control.

Recognise that because you are stressed you won't feel like using a stress management technique. That's the irony. The time you need them the most is the time you'll feel least like using them. That's why you must make Every Day Count. It will help you develop the stress coping habits you need.

There are courses available in all of these fightback techniques. The 'how to' explanations that follow will provide all you need to get you scoring pressure points and reversing stress trends. If you feel like you need more information, sign up for a short course.

When stress happens in your life, I recommend these 5 techniques: massage, spa, progressive muscle contraction and relaxation, mental imagery, and meditation.

MASSAGE

Massage is like exercise without the sweat. It's also very therapeutic, soothing and enjoyable. Spending time with a professional masseur is ideal; however, you can still perform a worthwhile massage even if you are not an expert.

Physically, massage improves blood flow to the areas being stimulated. When blood flow is increased, oxygen supply is enhanced and waste disposal is improved. Massage can be self- or partner-performed.

There are many types of massage techniques. The simplest is to take a fold of skin in between your thumb and forefinger. Use both hands at once so that you have two separate skin folds in your hands. Start at the base of the skin fold. Gently roll the skin fold between your thumb and finger as you work up and away from the body to the part of the skin fold you have pulled away from the body. Gently release the skin and grasp two new skin folds. Repeat the process as you cover the desired areas.

Another technique is to simply use the palms of your hands in a circular motion to soothe and relax an area. Use the heels of your hands or your thumbs when you want to apply more pressure. The rapid dual-hand karate chop technique known as 'petrissage' looks impressive but is better left to the experts.

The neck, shoulders, upper back and arms are all ideal massage sites, though individual preferences will determine exactly where you receive your massage. When you are being massaged you will assist the process and maximise the gains if you control your breathing with regular, deep inhalations and exhalations. Don't tense up when the masseur hits a tender spot. Try to relax and enjoy the experience. Just 20 minutes is enough to earn you a full day's quota of pressure points.

Massage isn't only a fightback technique. It can also be a vital preventative tool. Perhaps you could schedule time for one professional massage once each week, negotiate a deal with your partner for a second 20-minute amateur massage once each week and self-massage for 20 minutes once each week. Follow this schedule and already you will be scoring your 4 pressure points on 3 days per week.

SPA

If massage is exercise without sweat, spa is massage with the masseur. The very act of taking time for a spa bath is a victory against the tyranny of time. Apart from the jinx

147

that immersing yourself in warm water is a surefire way to make the phone ring, baths and spas create a great feeling of security and serenity. Try to promote this mindset and you will maximise the therapeutic value of the time you spend 'in hydro'. Just remember to take the phone off the hook first.

Enjoying a spa is more than psychologically beneficial. There are well-documented physical benefits as well. The jets of water hitting your shoulders and back have a similar effect to a pair of hands massaging your skin. Baths are good, spas are better.

Professional sportspeople have been using spas for decades as a rehabilitative and recuperative measure after hard training or matches. Muscle microtrauma is a term used to describe the thousands of tiny, microscopic muscle tears that occur not only during active sports participation, but as part of day-to-day life. Massage and spa are excellent means of repairing this muscle microtrauma.

Some people are reluctant to use public spa pools, and rightly so. Unless you have absolute faith in the people who maintain the water quality of the spa pool and you can guarantee that they monitor this water quality daily, don't use that spa. If you are forced to use public spa pools, never put your head under water and avoid the spa whenever you have any cuts or grazes. Spas are great. They are also great havens for germs and bacteria.

The best spa is the one you fill with warm water just before you use it, and drain when you are finished. A standard bathtub can be easily converted into a spa by using a portable pump designed specifically for this purpose. Take the time to spend 20 relaxing minutes in a spa bath at least once a week. It's a passive, restful and luxurious way to redeem the effects of stress and earn yourself 1 point for every 5 minutes you're soaking.

PROGRESSIVE MUSCLE CONTRACTION AND RELAXATION

You may think of massage and spa as being passive stress busters because the work is done for you. However, they will only be fully effective when you contribute by being in the right frame of mind.

One means of developing the right frame of mind is through the use of a technique known as progressive muscle contraction and relaxation. This technique works on the principle that you have to create tension before you can release tension. You squeeze your muscles and then you relax them. Think of a rubber band. If you stretch the band tightly for a few seconds and then release the tension, it relaxes beyond its starting position. When you tightly contract your muscles for a few seconds and then release that tension, your muscles will relax past their initial level. This technique overrides muscle tone and allows you to reach a degree of physical relaxation you will not normally achieve.

It is preferable to start with your toes and progressively work upward along your body. If you can find somewhere private, the best position is to lie on your back or recline in a chair. Body parts touching each other should be kept to a minimum. Spread your legs slightly and keep your arms by your sides rather than draped across your body. Keep your hands unclenched for the moment, fingers separated, your eyes closed and your mouth open.

The most difficult aspect of the technique to master is to keep breathing. It's as natural to want to hold your breath when you tense as it is for a novice golfer to slice the ball or for a learning netball player to take too many steps. You must keep breathing to allow the tension to ease. It may not feel natural to breathe in and out as you tense and hold a body part, but this is exactly what you need to do.

Here's a 20-minute relaxation program that will earn you 4 pressure points. Start with a 2-minute breathing cycle; in for a count of 3, hold for a count of 3 and exhale for a count of 3. Next, establish a pattern of 'in for a count of 3 and out for a count of 3' without any pause or interim holding of breath. Keep this going for the next 2 minutes. You are now at the start of the fifth minute. No matter what else happens, stay with the 'in–2–3–out–2–3' breathing schedule until you complete the entire 20-minute session.

Dig your heels into the carpet as hard as you can. Hold them there until your legs start to shake. Don't set a period because as soon as you start to count, you'll upset your breathing rhythm. It might be as little as 5 seconds or as long as 20 seconds. You'll find your own level. Slowly release the pressure. Your heels will feel like they want to lift off the ground. This is the start of the real relaxation process.

Wait through 2 full inhalations and exhalations before the next contraction, which is to curl up your toes. Think of the tightest fitting school shoes you ever had, shrink them another 3 sizes and mentally try to fit your toes inside. Hold them there in that cramped, painful state as long as you can manage and imagine your toes slowly breaking through the shoes into glorious freedom. Another 2 breath cycles before progressing.

Now it's your calves. Try to tense your entire lower leg while the rest of your body stays relaxed. Remember to maintain the all important breathing rhythm. Hold until the sensation is about to deteriorate from discomfort to pain, then slowly release. You'll really start to feel how your muscles relax past the state they were in before you started. You can add to the experience by imagining the tension dripping out of your legs in the relaxation phase.

Repeat the exercise with your thighs. You can combine the front and back of your thighs at the same time, though it's preferable to separate the quadriceps at the front of your thigh and the hamstrings at the rear if you have the ability and the time to do so. Remember that this is earning you a point for every 5 minutes you invest, so take your time.

Continue with the abdomen, lower back, shoulders and arms in respective order. Each body part takes around 60 seconds by the time you stress, relax and wait for 2 full breath cycles before continuing.

When you get to your hands, make tight fists as if you were Superman trying to squeeze a diamond out of a piece of coal. You will have to concentrate hard to prevent yourself from tensing other body parts and holding your breath. Exaggerate the relaxing phase by slowly unclenching your fists. You may actually experience some resistance, as if your fingers don't want to open out, though when you do manage to prise them apart you won't have to imagine the tension dripping out of your fingers: it will be reality. Making a fist is one of the classic postures for tension and aggression. If you can make a fist without tensing your entire body, you will have developed another vital skill in the war against the stress response.

To complete the progressive contraction and relaxation exercise you need to tense and relax your neck and finally your facial muscles. To do this you clench your teeth, furrow your brow and contort your cheeks. Just pray no one takes a photo! It feels weird the first time, but so do many things we quickly acquire tastes for. We carry a lot of tension in our facial muscles and the feeling of releasing this tension, especially when you have already prepared the rest of your body, is very worthwhile. Try it, you'll enjoy it.

The entire process should take you around 20 minutes. That's your 4 pressure points earned for today.

MENTAL IMAGERY

Some techniques will suit your persona more than others will. If you are an imaginative or creative person, you will find mental imagery as natural as daydreaming. It's a technique based on changing your focus from your conscious mind to your subconscious mind.

Test cricketer Mark Waugh once took the hardest catch of his life and dropped the easiest catch of his life within 5 minutes. The hardest catch was a 'blinder'. The ball was edged from a fast bowler and deflected away from where Mark was fielding. He dived full length to his left and thrust out one hand to complete what seemed like an impossible take. It all happened so quickly that you had to watch the slow motion replay 2 or 3 times to really work out what had actually happened. There was certainly no time for conscious thought from Mark's point of view. It was a combination of great skill, reflexes and years of training that enabled him to pull up an incredible sporting feat.

During the very next over, Mark was fielding close in to the batsman who tried to hook a short pitch ball from a slow bowler. The ball caught the top edge of the bat and ballooned 10 metres or so up in the air. Mark was comfortably positioned under the ball and he had plenty of time to watch it gently lob into his hands. On a scale of 1 to 10, the catch Mark had just taken was a 10, and this was a simple 1. It was what they call a 'snack,' but unbelievably, Mark dropped the ball.

I'm surmising that the difference between taking the hard catch and dropping the easy catch was Mark's mindset. In the first case, there was no conscious thought;

it was a purely subconscious, reflex action. In the second case, he had time to think. He had time to wonder whether or not he would make the catch, time to consider how he was on television and being watched by millions of people, time to think about how much his team needed this wicket and time to hear the heckling fans in the stands.

Our conscious mind is both friend and foe. It enables us to think and we would never want to lose this. It also gives us the chance to think too much. The conscious mind is the one telling us to be achievers, make the deadline, accumulate more money and push ourselves onward and upward. Our conscious mind is the one vasoconstricting our blood vessels and elevating our pulse rate.

Our subconscious mind doesn't tell us to think anything because it operates on a level without thoughts we recognise or are aware of. It sends signals to our muscles to relax so our blood vessels can vasodilate and our pulse rate can slow down. We must get our subconscious mind into the action when we are awake, not just when we are asleep.

Mental imagery is about leaving the world behind for a while and escaping to your imagination, to your subconscious mind. Start with your 2 minutes of breathing: in for 3, hold for 3 and out for 3.

From here on in you have to let it happen rather than make it happen. Close your eyes or focus on a spot until it ceases to dominate your vision. You will still see the spot, though you are aware of other things as well.

Next you try to think of yourself being in a favourite place, but before you do, you have to eliminate the baggage. Any worries or concerns you have should be thought of as small black boxes. Imagine yourself walking out of a building through a series of doors that automatically slide open as you approach them. Just before each door there is a rubbish bin with its lid open, inviting you to throw away your troubles. In your mind's eye, as you are walking out of this building, wrap your trouble box in a blue-green cloth and drop it in the bin as you walk past. The bin lid snaps shut, the door shuts behind you and the trouble is gone. As you approach the next doorway, get rid of another trouble. Walk through as many doors as you need to until all your troubles are gone, at least metaphorically.

When you walk through the last door, you enter your special place. This may be anywhere from a beach to a bed. You can be in a group or alone, it can be noisy or quiet, in colour or mono. You don't have to imagine a gently stream flowing by or a white light approaching. You can still be conscious of the fact that you are imagining something other than it being reality. Don't try to fathom your mind. It's like trying to solve a Rubic's cube when you only have 2 of the 4 sides to work with.

Just imagine having a good time and keep the dream going. You probably won't get so involved that you lose track of time. If you do, fantastic; if you don't, keep returning to your fantasy until you've been in dreamland for at least 15 minutes. If you make it for 20 minutes, you will have earned your 4 stress points today. You can use this technique at the office, at home, even on public transport, but please, not while you are driving!

Mental imagery is a skill and like all skills it needs practice. Try it today. Go to dreamworld at least once each week. When you use massage, hydrotherapy, muscle contractions and imagery you are developing a strong range of weapons in your fightback against when stress happens.

MEDITATION

It's hard to do meditation justice in a few lines. The most powerful thing I can write about meditation is that you can do it. Doing a course is the ideal; trying it for yourself is a great start.

A friend of mine went on a 9-day meditation retreat where he spoke only to an instructor once a day and spent the majority of his waking hours in meditation. By the end of the program he was travelling in his mind's eye. He was 'travelling' inside his body as if he was a microscopic camera. He experienced actually being a breath, being inhaled into his own lungs and then exhaled up through his windpipe and out through his mouth and nose. This is quite dangerous and something my friend wisely stopped straight away and returned his thoughts to a more conscious plane. It does show, however, just how powerful meditation is. At the deeper levels of meditation, people can have incredible experiences.

At our level we are simply looking to reach a new state of thought. It's not the control of thought or the blocking of thought; it's the absence of thought.

You are trying to reach a place in your mind where you simply exist, you are there, you know you are there, but your conscious mind isn't registering that you are there. Sounds as if I've been inhaling too much incense, I know, but that is exactly what it feels like. Part of you knows that you are lying on your back in a dark room with soft music on at the same time as a large part of you becomes dormant. You are not really thinking anything, you don't have a sense of heightened smell or hearing, you are just there. It's not the blocking of thoughts; it's the absence of thoughts.

155

How you get there takes trial and error. You can sit cross-legged in the lotus position, recline in a chair or lie comfortably without too many body parts touching. You'll know if the lotus is right for you within the first minute. It either feels great or it gives you cramps along your entire lower body. It gives me cramps, so I just lie on my back.

You can fixate on one spot or you can use mental imagery or muscular contractions and relaxation to help you reach the desired state of relaxation. As they say in the hair commercials, it won't happen overnight, but yes, it will happen. My best estimate is that it will take you between 1 and 4 hours before you realise for the first time that you have been meditating. You won't realise you've done it until it's over and your conscious mind registers where you have been.

Don't try too hard; you can't make it happen, you have to allow it to happen. If you spend the time, you will get the result. People who are skilled at meditation can reach the state they want within a couple of minutes. They can even do a shallow meditation for a few seconds to clear their mind during a busy day. If you are an enthusiastic novice like myself, you are better off allocating at least 20 minutes per session. You earn 4 stress points and it's a good time compromise between being too rushed and too ambitious while your meditation skills are developing.

Meditation may not be something you've ever given much serious thought to. It's really no different from knowing the home keys on a typewriter and being able to type at a basic level or knock a golf ball around a course. It's a skill that we can all develop to a greater or lesser extent. There are always going to be faster typists and better golfers, but it doesn't stop the rest of us having a go and getting a reward for our efforts.

A FINAL WORD ON STRESS

Think positive. There is no way you can say 'think positive' without sounding trite, but it is perhaps the truest of all truisms. If the day sends you lemons, make lemonade. Whatever way you look at your predicament, a half-full glass seems to hold more than a half-empty one and a positive frame of mind sends positive, healthy signals to our physical being.

Fighting stress takes time and practice. It won't always work for you first time. Please keep at it because you only run out of chances when you stop taking them.

Former West Indian opening batsman Desmond Haynes had a simple 3-word philosophy about life which he wore inscribed on a gold neck chain. Desmond may not have to cope with the stress of corporate life but he was facing the potential stress of the fastest bowlers in the world as his 9 to 5 job. His credo says a lot in just 3 words 'Live – Laugh – Love'. Good advice Des.

What do I do now?

Now that you know all about how to score food, exercise and pressure points, it's time to commence a 2-week program trial. During this period you will discover whether 25 food choices each day is right for you and you will find that some stress prevention and coping devices work better for you than others.

Use the next 2 weeks to adjust yourself to the program and adjust the program to you:

1 Count and score your daily food choices. Aim for a net daily score of 12 points from 25 food choices. Be aware of keeping the fat content of the food you eat during the course of the day to between 40 and 50 grams.

2 Score all the exercise you do regardless of the intensity, on the basis of 1 point for every 15 minutes invested. Aim for 1 hour (4 points) of exercise on 4 days each week.

3 Practise counting pressure points every day over the next fortnight. Score 1 point each time you use a technique to block a stress stimulus, even if it only takes you a matter of seconds to do so. Score points for the relaxation and rehabilitation activities that you use on the basis of 1 point for every 2 minutes. Aim for 4 points every day, including weekends.

4 Read Chapter 9 and Appendix 2 to extend your knowledge of what foods rate as +, 0 and – options.

5 Record your 2-week trial in the space provided in the trial diary (see Appendix 3).

6 Think about the 7 daily, weekly and monthly rewards that you are going to commit to building into your program. You have 2 weeks to get these organised before you start the program in earnest.

7 Mentally prepare yourself to begin the full program after your 2-week trial.

It's said that 'a dream is a goal with a deadline'. It's time for action now.

9

FAST FOOD FIGURES

'Genius is in the details.'

CENTRAL INTELLIGENCE AGENCY TRAINING EDICT

EXCEPTIONAL ALES

We have rated the majority of common foodstuffs and drinks as either +1, 0 or −1. Your challenge is to include enough +1 choices in your diet each day to build up a food score of 12 points. This is the idea of Every Day Counts.

Most foods and drinks always rate positively, neutrally or negatively, regardless of how many times you choose them on a given day. Cooked potato chips are always −1 because of their high fat content. Apples are always +1 because they are low in fat and high in carbohydrate. Of course too much of any food or drink could be toxic. No one is recommending that you should eat 8 apples a day to generate a positive food score. This would be unrealistic and outside the spirit of the system.

There are 5 exceptions to the rule that all common food and drink choices are rated as +1, 0 or −1. These exceptions normally rate as a positive point when chosen once or twice, but then rate negatively if chosen again that day. Whenever there is an exception or an additional explanation is provided, you will find this information under the *Comments* heading in the tables of Appendix 2: Food lists. The five exceptions are:

Alcohol On a daily basis, your first 10 ounces of beer or wine (red or white) or your first shot of spirits counts as +1. Alcohol has legitimate nutritional, medicinal and therapeutic value. Happy days! Your second for the day also rates as +1!

Before you start the party, you should know that any and all additional drinks you have on that day rate as −1. The world might look like a better place after a few more drinks, but alcohol is a depressant and too much will send your mood, as well as your daily points score, heading in the wrong direction. Please remember that your third drink is a −1, it is not a 0.

Fruit juice Your first 2 fruit juice drinks each day also rate as +1. Fresh juice is a good food choice, though fruit itself is better. A glass of orange juice may take the fluid of 5 or 6 oranges to make. Unfortunately the fibre and vitamin rich pulp is lost to you when you choose the juice option. Every orange contains a lot of natural sugar, called fructose. Two orange juice drinks have the equivalent sugar content of 10 to 12 actual oranges.

That's okay, but if you have 5 ojs, that would be the equivalent of the juice from 30 oranges in one day. That's too many. A high intake of sugar like this is begging your liver to store some of the excess, and you know how the excess is stored. That's right, as fat! You can't put on weight by eating too many vegetables, but you can put on weight by eating too much fruit. It's not only oranges, it's all fruit. It's also tough on your sugar regulation system to have so much coming in each day. That's why your first two juices of the day are +1 and after that they are −1.

Sports drinks These drinks have no fat content but can be 8% or more carbohydrate. Too much carbohydrate in your daily intake will lead to conversion to fat and storage. It's almost a de facto means of taking in hidden fat. For this reason, while your first 2 sports drinks for the day hold +1 ratings, third and subsequent sports drinks are negative.

Tea and coffee Caffeine is a stimulant and a positive one when taken in moderation. It's also addictive and has a number of negative side-effects when used in high dosages. A little is okay though we definitely don't want too much coming in every day. There's also the matter of what's taken in with each cup, especially if you're partial to a couple of spoonfuls of sugar, a dollop of full-cream milk and maybe a couple of sweet biscuits. Your first 2 teas or coffees (or one of each) for the day rate as +1, as long as it's no more than 'white with one'. After that it's all downhill. Your third and subsequent teas or coffees (including decaf) each day rate as –1. Herbal teas always count as +1.

Notice the trend? These 4 exceptions are positive for the first 2 choices and then negative for the rest of the day. They are also all drinks. You may have deduced that variation and moderation (except in the case of water, which is positive for the first 8 glasses and then rates a 0 for every additional glass) are the keys to the right type of fluid intake. There are no foods or drinks that start off being negative and then become positive from the third choice onward. It just doesn't work like that.

Eggs The fifth exception is eggs. Eggs are the only food exception. Your first 2 eggs for the *week* are +1 choices; after that they are –1 choices. Egg yolks are high in fat and packed with cholesterol. Have as many egg whites as you like. They are full of protein and definite +1 choices. It is the egg yolks that are the problem so please limit these.

These are the only 5 exceptions to the rule that choices are always +1, 0 or −1. The fact that 4 of the 5 are drinks (alcohol, juice, sports drink, and tea or coffee) makes these exceptions easy to remember and easy to manage.

EAT, DRINK AND BE WARY

USING THE FOOD LISTS
The food lists in Appendix 2 are in 2 forms. The first section lists foods according to type, for example fruits, breads, meats and so on. This list includes the fat content of each food choice in grams, per 100 grams by weight. These figures will help you to measure your fat intake and keep the total for the day to between 40 and 50 grams. The second section lists food and drink choices in alphabetical order, plus the same information.

When you are looking for a specific food, try the alphabetical listings first. When you want to compare how foods rate with others of a similar nature, for example how an apple compares with a banana, you'll find the group listings more beneficial.

The fat content is listed in grams per 100 grams unless specified otherwise. With breads, for example, we have listed the fat content per slice, rather than per 100 grams. This will make it easier for you to calculate your grams of fat intake on an ongoing basis.

It is important to be aware that fat content will vary according to the quality of the original food, the method of cooking and any additives or condiments used. Use these tables as a guide to control daily fat intake and calculate your daily food score.

What do I do now?
Keep working through your 2-week trial period.

1 Count and score your daily food choices.
2 Score your exercise efforts on 4 days each week during the trial.
3 Score pressure points each day.
4 Keep recording your trial scores in the space provided in the trial diary (see Appendix 3).
5 Settle on your daily, weekly and monthly rewards.
6 Read Chapters 10 and 11 for additional exercise ideas and an 'extra edge' before you make a final commitment.

Special thanks to Matt Hornsby, Susie Parker, Lorna Garden and the Australian Nutrition Foundation for their help in preparing this chapter and the food lists.

10

PERSONAL BEST: TRAINING FOR FITNESS

'Don't wait for your ship to come in, swim out to it.'

STRENGTH AND STAMINA

Every Day Counts will keep you healthy and well. Preparing yourself for competitive sport or peak athletic performance is another matter. This chapter is designed for people who are looking for this extra dimension in their training.

The conditioning programs detailed in this chapter won't score you any more exercise points than gentle walking or working in the garden; it's still 1 point for every 15 minutes when you are counting every day. The primary principle of Every Day Counts is about getting well. This chapter goes one step further: it is about getting fit.

To achieve real fitness, you must develop both stamina and strength.

STAMINA SECRETS

The first 'S' component of fitness is stamina.

Stamina is also known as aerobic fitness, cardiovascular fitness, cardio-respiratory fitness, endurance and lactate tolerance. All these terms basically describe the same parametre. Stamina is heart and lung fitness. It is the ability to keep supplying the required amounts of oxygen to the muscles in an efficient manner.

Our muscles need oxygen to work. Oxygen, along with glycogen (digested food), is the fuel that enables our muscles to contract, therefore allowing us to move. Our skeleton is like a puppet. Our muscles are the strings that move the skeleton, and our brain and nervous system are the puppet masters. The heart pumps the blood, and the blood carries the oxygen and glycogen around the body to the muscles.

If you're riding a bike, a greater quantity of blood is directed to the legs because it's the leg muscles doing the majority of the work. If you're performing biceps curls, more blood is distributed to the upper body to keep up the supply of glycogen and oxygen to this region. This is called preferential blood flow.

The final link in the chain is the lungs. The lungs inhale air and transfer oxygen into the bloodstream in exchange for the used-up, stale air containing carbon dioxide. The stale air is promptly exhaled before we again draw in a new supply of fresh, oxygen-rich air.

Stamina is simply a measure of how efficiently this integrated system works. It's how efficiently you inhale air, have oxygen ready for the blood to pick up, and how efficient your heart is in transporting the oxygen once it's reached the bloodstream. The performance of the muscles themselves is also a factor though we'll deal with that independently when we get to the strength section.

THE HUMAN SPEEDO

The most reliable means of measuring your stamina training is to use a heart-rate monitor. Monitoring heart rates as a guide to training output and intensity is not a new concept, but as a means of choosing the right level for you to train at, heart-rate monitors are without doubt the best 'fitness purchase' you could ever make.

It's now the rule rather than the exception to use a heart-rate monitor instead of relying on manually 'finger felt' heart rates in all modes of training. If you're not using electronic monitoring, you really are being left behind. Monitoring your heart rate during exercise is like checking your tachometer while driving a car. It's important to know how many 'revs' your engine is doing.

The classic rule of thumb is that your maximum heart rate is likely to be 220 beats less your age. According to this rule, a 40-year-old is likely to have a maximum heart rate of around 180 beats per minute (220 – 40 = 180). Traditional exercise methodology is to then calculate 70% of your predicted maximum to determine how hard you should be training. Seventy per cent of 180 beats per minute equals 126 beats per minute. Therefore, the traditional advice was for all 40-year-olds to exercise at this level to improve their stamina.

If only it was that simple! People are individuals and in reality their maximum heart rates vary just as much as their shapes, size and looks. There can be variations of up to 30 beats either way from this very general estimate of heart-rate maximums. A 40-year-old may have a maximum heart rate of only 150 beats per minute, not the 180 beats per minute predicted on the basis of age only.

When a 40 year old works out at 126 beats per minute and his or her maximum heart rate is only 150 beats per minute, the training load is over 85% of maximum. While this level of intensity is appropriate for elite athletic conditioning, for the average person it can be dangerous. It's like driving your car so hard the rev counter goes into the red zone. If you keep driving your car in the red zone it will overheat and your engine will eventually fail. It's the same thing with your human engine!

Heart-rate monitors are certainly more accurate than manually measuring heart rates. Leading brand 'Polar', has been independently tested and proven to be within 1 beat per minute of an electrocardiogram heart rate reading at intensities of up to 180 beats per minute. This is accurate! Heart-rate monitors eliminate the guesswork.

Just because you have a heart-rate monitor, however, you have no guarantee of working out at the right level. You will know how fast your heart is beating, but is this too fast, too slow or just right? The best way to establish your true, individual heart-rate training range is to start with the 220-minus-your-age guide and match this to a perceived level of exertion of 7 out of 10 on your own personal scale. Don't be a prisoner to any one particular number. If you are 50 years of age, your predicted maximum heart rate will be 170 beats per minute. Seventy per cent of your maximum is 119 beats per minute. If you reach this level and it feels very comfortable, perhaps a 5 out of 10 on your subjective perceived exertion scale, increase your training heart rate by 5 beats and reassess.

It will take you only a few exercise sessions to determine the right training heart rate for you as an individual. This is the real benefit of heart-rate monitoring. The monitor allows you to establish exactly what your optimum level is. Once you know the right figures, the monitor will help you stay in the right training zone.

What sort of exercise are heart-rate monitors used for? There are literally no restrictions. Running, cycling, walking and circuit training are the most popular applications, though the monitors are fully functional in water and so can be used for swimming and other aqua training. They have been trialled in contact sports such as Australian Rules football, though there is the chance of damage to the transmitter through physical contact. In these instances, the 'watch' or wrist receiver is normally not worn. Rather, the heart-rate data is stored in the transmitter and later downloaded into a computer for analysis.

There are no wires connecting the transmitter chest strap and the receiver wrist 'watch'. These units are not like the old 'ear plug' or 'chest strap to gauge' models. A signal is sent from the chest strap through the air to the receiver. The receiver is usually worn as a watch though it can be held by the coach or training partner as long as they stay within a range of a couple of metres. Women are at no disadvantage when wearing a monitor because of their breasts. The chest strap can be comfortably worn below the breasts without any loss of accuracy in the readings.

Many monitors have in-built alarms that can be preset so that if your heart rate falls below or exceeds your desired heart-rate range, a warning buzzer sounds. You can adjust your intensity immediately to provide a safe and efficient workout.

WHY USE A HEART-RATE MONITOR?

Heart monitors work. They act as a personal tachometer! Never before have we had such a practical and affordable means of constant feedback on how we are coping with exercise. No longer do we need to rely on subjective feelings or someone else's observations. Heart-rate monitors tell us exactly how our body is responding. This provides an added degree of safety as it protects us from the possibility of working too hard in order to gain a training effect.

These monitors really are the best thing that's happened in sports science this century! They have done to fitness training what word processors have done to writing letters, what dishwashers have done to cleaning up and what remote controls have done to watching television. But while these trappings of modern living have all made our life more sedentary, the beauty of heart-rate monitors is that they encourage the opposite. They are a tool that encourages activity rather than inactivity.

WHERE YOU'RE AT

Use your monitor to measure your current level of stamina. If you cannot gain access to a heart-rate monitor, you can still try this simple test. It's called the Queen's College step test and it is easy and quick to administer. It will give you a guide to your level of stamina comparative to others.

You'll need a bench or step that is 40 centimetres in height. Starting with both feet on the floor, step up one foot at a time onto the step and then down again to the floor. You should complete 22 step ups (up-up-down-down) per minute for 3 minutes. When the 3 minutes is up, sit quietly for 15 seconds and watch your heart-rate response. If you are working without a monitor use the 15 seconds to find your pulse. Count your heartbeats for the next 30 seconds, then double the number to calculate your heart rate for a minute. The lower your pulse rate, the fitter you are. Compare your result to the percentile table below. The more towards the bottom of the table you are, the quicker your recovery has been and the fitter you are. As an example, a woman's heart rate of 148 beats per minute falls in the ninetieth percentile which means that only 10% of women would have a heart rate this low after the step-up test.

Only do this test to measure your fitness if you already exercise regularly and you believe you have at least a basic level of fitness. This is not a way to get fit; it's a measure of how fit you are. It's quite demanding, even though it lasts for only 3 minutes. If you are in doubt about how to measure your fitness, start with the 5-minute test that is explained after this table. How will you rate?

Percentile	Male heart rate	Female heart rate
5	184	196
10	178	184
15	176	182
20	172	180
25	168	176
30	166	172
35	164	171
40	162	170
45	160	168
50	156	166
55	154	164
60	152	163
65	149	162
70	148	160
75	144	158
80	140	156
85	136	152
90	128	148
95	124	140
100	120	128

There is another, more gentle test that you may find more appropriate if you don't think you are quite up to the 3-minute step test. Please don't just read about it, do it. All you have to do is walk, jog or run as far as you can in 5 minutes. Don't push past the level of slight discomfort. Six or seven out of 10 on your perceived exertion scale is about right.

It is of no value for you to try harder at this stage. You will not get fitter by pushing too much. Take note of the distance you cover in the 5 minutes. You don't have to know your actual distance in metres or kilometres, just as long as you remember your distance with a marker, a tree or lamp-post, or anything that you will remember. This is your base.

Most new trainers will cover between 500 metres and 1.5 kilometres in the 5-minute test. Let's assume that you travelled exactly 1 kilometre in the 5-minute time trial and you have an aim of improving your performance by 10%, through 3 weeks of training. Your target on day 21 will be to cover 1100 metres in the 5-minute test.

DOWN TO BUSINESS

The training program that follows is designed for someone who achieved approximately 1000 metres in his or her initial 5-minute time trial. If you cover less than 1000 metres in your 5-minute time trial, start with more moderate sessions, then still build up with similar increments.

If you are already more advanced and can travel more than 1000 metres in 5 minutes, you will have to start with more challenging sessions and again build the difficulty over the 3-week training period.

The program combines the use of interval and overdistance training. I hope you enjoy it.

Day 1   5-minute time trial. The distance covered is assumed to be exactly 1000 metres.

Day 2   Slow 5-kilometre walk or run. Don't be concerned with time, finish the distance even if you have to stop and rest for a time.

Day 3   Stretch for 15 minutes following a 20-minute recuperation walk. Please don't run today.

Day 4   15-minute warm-up walk or run, then 10 x 250 metre walk or run throughs at about two-thirds of your top pace. Recover by jogging (or walking more slowly) half-way back to the start (125 metres) and walking (or walking very slowly) the rest of the way. If you are running, it should take you about 45 seconds for each run through and about 2 minutes for each jog/walk back. This gives you a work to rest ratio of 1:3. This is your target. If you get back to the start before 2 minutes, rest until the 2-minute mark before starting your next run through. Remember you are doing 10 walk or run throughs so don't try for any speed records on the first 2 or 3. Professional athletes always keep to the pre-designed schedule for that day so don't fall into the trap of too fast-too soon.

Day 5   20-minute walk or run. The first 5 minutes are slow, the next 10 minutes are at 70% effort and the final 5 minutes are as slow and relaxed as the first 5. Finish with a slow routine of stretching. Hold each stretch position for at least 5 seconds.

Day 6   Rest.

Day 7   Warm up with a slow walk or jog and a thorough stretch. Your aim today is to walk or run solidly for 20 minutes. An 'out and back' (see our oddball workouts in Chapter 6) course can be used simply by walking or running as far as you can in 10 minutes, then turning around and trying to make it back to the start in the next 10 minutes. You are aiming for maximum distance, though it is still advisable to keep something in reserve. Remind yourself of that perceived level of exertion of 7 out of 10. If you have a monitor, don't exceed your target heart rate. At your current level, there is little or no physiological advantage in running at 90% capacity as compared to 70% capacity. We must get through this 21-day program without injury to enjoy its full benefits. Avoid the temptation of pushing yourself too hard at this stage. That will come later!

Day 8   Today is an easy day. A long, slow walk of between 50 and 60 minutes is your sole task.

Day 9   Repeat Day 4 but with an extra 5 repetitions of your walk or run throughs. The timing remains the same, 45 seconds if you are doing run throughs and 2 minutes for the recovery. Fifteen repetitions, then a slow jog and stretch to cool down.

Day 10   Rest.

Day 11   More interval work today. Your target is 20 x 50 to 80 metre strides 'on the minute'. If you are walking, your stride distance is 50 metres. If you are running, your stride distance is 80 metres. This is your speed work. Each walk or run through will take you about 14 seconds, which leaves you 46 seconds to slow down, turnaround and walk or jog back to the start. This is what 'on the minute' means. You may start to feel that your strides are getting slower and your recoveries are getting faster, just to keep on the schedule of getting back in time for the next stride through on the minute. A slow 10-minute walk and stretch finishes your session for the day.

Day 12   Rest.

Day 13   We now move back into overdistance training. Today's session is 40 minutes of slow tempo walking, running or run/walking. Don't be overly concerned if you have to stop, though it is preferable to keep your pace as constant as possible. You're better off averaging 6-minute running kilometres or 9-minute walking kilometres rather than running for some of the time at a furious pace and other times at a dawdle. Finish with a good lower back and groin stretch.

Day 14 Today is a repeat of Day 7. After warming up it's a 20-minute walk or run, as far as you can from the start in 10 minutes and then back to the start (hopefully) in the next 10 minutes.

Day 15 Repeat yesterday's session. This will give you an indication of your progress. You should be within 50 metres of yesterday's performance level, both in the 10-minute 'out' mark and in the 10-minute 'return'. If you are not within this range, it's time to temporarily back off as you are struggling to recover between sessions. Rest for the next 2 days, then recommence the program from Day 1.

If you are within the recommended range of 50 metres from yesterday's performance, stick with the last few days of the program.

Day 16 Rest.

Day 17 This is your last interval session designed to build speed: 10 x 250 walk or run throughs at a comfortable speed. Don't think you have to race, just keep an even tempo, 90 seconds recovery between each stride through. 5-minute cool down jog and a full stretch afterwards.

Day 18 You're now into your taper. An easy, relaxed 20-minute walk or run today. Don't measure your distance or heart rate; just use the session to rid your body of the accumulated wastes from yesterday's harder lactate work.

Day 19 20-minute slow walk and stretch.

Day 20 Rest and mental rehearsal (earn pressure points today by dreaming of a good performance) for tomorrow's 5-minute time trial.

Day 21 Second test. Target of 1100 metres in 5 minutes.

This program works to improve your stamina by progressively increasing the intensity of the workouts. This 21-day program can be used in conjunction with the Every Day Counts system by allocating yourself 1 exercise point for every 15 minutes on any of the 4 exercise days in any given week.

STRENGTH SECRETS

The second 'S' component of fitness is strength. The following information is designed to help you to start your own strength-building program.

Which of the following do you believe is the better test of strength? The maximum amount you can lift in a bench press exercise in a single all out effort? Or the maximum number of push ups you can do before your muscles give out on you and you have to rest? The answer is that they really indicate different types of strength. The maximum bench press measures explosive strength or power while the push ups test measures your muscular endurance. There is quite a big difference between 'power strength' and 'endurance strength' and it is difficult and inefficient to try to improve both at the same time. A disadvantage of maximum bench press and other maximum lifts is that they are potentially dangerous for someone who has previously been untrained or undertrained.

Many athletes and even some fitness trainers never really develop a working understanding of strength in its dual forms. If you'd like to get stronger, the ideal is to first develop a base of muscular endurance. This means building a muscular endurance foundation through relatively light levels of resistance. This is what our program is going to work on. The results will be increased strength, tone and muscular definition. You'll look and feel better.

The training principle of progressive overload is very applicable when working to develop endurance strength. Improvements of up to 20% are often made in the first month of graduated training.

Our basic unit of reference will be poundage or kilograms per session. This is the total amount you lift or shift during your workouts. Each workout is designed to take 60 minutes and earn you 4 exercise points as you make Every Day Count. We will be using 6 basic core exercises and a routine of 4 sets on each of these exercises. The repetitions making up each set start with 8 and increase progressively to 12. Once you get to 12 repetitions, the resistance increases and the repetitions start again at 8. It's all laid out in the program that follows.

You will need to commit yourself to 3 'endurance strength' sessions per week. That leaves you only one other exercise day to keep up with your Every Day Counts requirements for the week. Please make that fourth session each week aerobic exercise so that you keep the balance between strength and stamina.

Start in session 1 doing 4 sets of 8 repetitions on each of the 6 exercises. That's a total of 32 reps of 6 exercises. This equals 192 lifts or exercises in all.

In the second session you do 2 sets of 8 and 2 sets of 9 of each exercise. That's 34 reps of each exercise and 204 reps in all. In the third session you do 4 sets of 9 for a grand total of 216 repetitions. The fourth session is 2 sets of 9 and 2 sets of 10 on each exercise. The fifth session requires you to do 4 sets of 10. You keep increasing in this manner until your ninth workout when your challenge is to do 4 sets of 12. This is equal to 48 repetitions of each exercise and 288 lifts in all. By the tenth workout, you will be ready to increase the resistance. Return to 4 sets of 8, though now with a heavier weight. Increase the resistance you are using by no more than 2.5 kilograms. Continue with the same sequence.

This is how it looks as a table:

Session	Sets	Repetitions	Resistance
1	4	8.8.8.8. (four sets of 8)	30 kg (example)
2	4	9.9.8.8.	30 kg
3	4	9.9.9.9.	30 kg
4	4	10.10.9.9.	30 kg
5	4	10.10.10.10.	30 kg
6	4	11.11.10.10.	30 kg
7	4	11.11.11.11.	30 kg
8	4	12.12.11.11.	30 kg
9	4	12.12.12.12.	30 kg
10	4	8.8.8.8.	32.5 kg
11	4	9.9.8.8	32.5 kg

This is how you progressively overload your muscles to improve endurance strength. It's not easy but it does work. You will find that you will reach plateaus where you cannot increase your reps each session and you may have to stay on the same level for a week or longer. Every weight trainer experiences these plateaus. You simply stay on that level until you are ready to progress. Don't be a prisoner to your program. It's a guide, not a prescription!

The hardest part is selecting your starting level. There is no reliable formula to help you. Some coaches advise the use of a percentage of maximum lifts. This creates a problem for beginners who may not have mastered correct technique and have little grounding in the sport of weight training. There is too great a risk of soreness and injury from attempting maximums without a training base in the first place. Percentages of maximum lifts are dangerous!

Each exercise described below comes with a conservative recommended starting weight. Use this for your first session and if you complete 4 sets of 8 repetitions with ease in your first session and suffer no soreness the following day, then skip 1 or 2 sessions to 4 sets of 10 for your next workout.

While you may feel you are under-exerting for a session or two, this is the safest and most effective way of quickly establishing your levels without the risk of injury and a potential break in your training. If you are going to make an error, make a conservative error. Conservative errors have no consequences. Ambitious errors cause injury. If you find the starting weights too demanding, reduce it by at least 25% and start again. The only person you are competing with is yourself.

The exercises that follow are presented with a gym option and a home option. The gym option will be more effective in improving your endurance strength. However, if you have no alternative other than to train at home, you will still considerably improve your endurance strength levels.

A calculation of the total kilograms lifted will monitor your improvement. This works as follows. If you lifted 4 sets of 8 repetitions of 30 kilograms on each exercise, you will have completed 32 repetitions multiplied by the 6 exercises, giving you a total of 192 lifts for the session. In each lift you shifted 30 kilograms for a total or 5760 kilograms for the session.

Only count successfully completed lifts and use your third session as your base. The first 2 sessions really are needed to set the levels of resistance that are appropriate to your current capabilities. Your aim in 6 weeks of training is to increase your total resistance lifted by 25%! Following through our example, if your total for session three is 5760 kilograms, your aim in session 20 will be 7188 kilograms. This is an increase of 25%. This will be well within your grasp if you follow the program.

You may find it necessary to keep a chart and, unless your are a maths whiz, the use of a calculator will be helpful. Please take the time to keep these records. They provide a tremendous source of motivation and objective assessment of your rate of improvement.

Exercises	Starting weight	Home option
1 Bench press	Male: 40 kg Female: 25kg	Push ups
2 Triceps push down	Male: 15 kg Female: 10 kg	Chair dips
3 Seated leg press	Male: 50 kg Female: 30 kg	Single leg squats
4 Abdominal crunches	Male: 10 kg Female: 5 kg	Abdominal crunches
5 Barbell biceps curls	Male: 20 kg Female: 10 kg	Incline chin ups with hands under chair or table and feet on floor
6 Lat pull down	Male: 35 kg Female: 20 kg	Isometric outward arm pushes in doorway. Push and hold for 20 seconds, relax for 5 seconds

HOLD STILL TO GAIN STRENGTH

There is an alternative means of improving your endurance strength. Not only does it not require equipment; it doesn't even require movement! It's called isometric training.

Isometric exercise occurs when muscles contract even though there is no movement. This creates a high degree of pressure and tension that is advantageous from a strength and conditioning point of view. There is, however, a warning for anyone who has high blood pressure or a limited background in strength training. The tension without movement causes an elevation in blood pressure. This is not desirable for hypertensive people. If you fit into this category of suffering from high blood pressure, low resistance 'isotonic' programs will better serve your needs. Isotonic exercise occurs when muscles shorten or lengthen as they contract. Movement always occurs as part of an isotonic contraction. There is no movement with an isometric contraction.

Holding a set position for 20 seconds, releasing for 5 seconds, then again holding for 20 seconds performs each isometric exercise. This takes 45 seconds. You then have 15 seconds to rest and be ready to begin the next exercise. Therefore, each time a full minute elapses you must be ready to start the next exercise.

Time (min)	Exercise	Description
0–1	Prayer push	Standing. Push your hands together in front of your chest, fingers pointing directly upward. Hold for 20 sec, release for 5 sec, push again for 20 sec. Exhale as you commence the push, inhale quickly and exhale again.
1–2	Monkey pull	As for the prayer push, but your hands form a finger (monkey) grip and pull outwards. You will feel your arms shake but there should be no deliberate give to either side.
2–3	Prayer push	Repeat.
3–4	Monkey pull	Repeat.

4–5	Behind the head push	Standing, hands behind your neck, fingers interlocked and palms flush against each other. To be in the correct position your hands should be pointing downward and your elbows upward. Use the system of 2 full exhalations and a rapid inhalation for each of the 20-second contractions when you push your hands hard in to each other. Allow yourself only 5 seconds between the 2 pushes.
5–6	Behind the head pull	Similar position but again use the monkey grip so that you can pull outward. It's important to keep your head up during this exercise as forward neck flexion can cause strain in that area. Keep looking up!
6–7	Behind the head push	Repeat.
7–8	Behind the head pull	Repeat.
8–9	Biceps curls	Sit on a solid chair, preferably one with arms. Place your hands, palms upwards under the arms of the chair or under a solid desk or table in front of you. Your back should be straight and you should be in a comfortable position as you lift upward with your hands. Once again there is no actual movement, but you will feel the pressure in the main muscle belly of the biceps.

9–10	Wrap hugs	Still seated in your chair, wrap your arms around the rear or backrest of the chair. If you can't join hands behind you with your palms facing away from the chair, the chair is too broad and should be replaced by a leaner model. Once in position, squeeze inward with your arms toward your body. You will feel the main workload being done by your chest, but your arms and shoulders will also benefit.
10–11	Biceps curls	Repeat.
11–12	Wrap hugs	Repeat.
12–13	Leg ins	Still in your chair, ensure your back is straight and your feet are touching the floor. Keep your knees slightly forward. Simply push your inner thighs together and hold. This is one exercise you may have difficulty in maintaining the contraction for a full 20 seconds so concentrate and keep at it if you feel the pressure of your contraction begin to wane.
13–14	Leg outs	Start as you would for the leg ins, but keep your legs slightly apart and rest your hands on the outside of your mid-thighs. This is a dual benefit exercise because you must push in with your hands as you push out with your thighs. The emphasis is on full effort but

		no movement, so only ease off if your legs are overpowering the resistance of your arms and hands.
14–15	Leg ins	Repeat.
15–16	Leg outs	Repeat.
16–17	Squats	Forget the chair for the last 4 minutes. Stand with your back against a wall, and then keep your back straight while you bend your knees and slide down until your thighs are as flat and parallel with the floor as possible. Hold the position. If you need more of a challenge than the 20 seconds, hold for 45 and press down against your thighs with your hands, or combine some chest and leg work by performing a squat and prayer push.
17–18	Toe raises	Stand away from the wall and work on your balance. Rise up onto both toes, right up as far as you can manage. Hold the position to develop the strength of your calf muscles. Once you are comfortable with the position, again add one of the upper body exercises like an overhead pull or push, but be conscious of breathing out through your contraction, quickly inhaling and breathing out again.
18–19	Squats	Repeat.
19–20	Toe raises	Repeat.

Isometrics provide an alternative way of developing some basic strength without investing too much time or money. This program earns exercise points at our standard rate of 1 point per 15 minutes even though there is no real movement. Isometrics are a unique case. They can also be used as a top-up program for travellers and people with very busy lifestyles. You can even do these exercises while you're waiting at traffic lights. Not a bad way to burn off the stress of the day.

SPEED SECRETS

A third fitness 'S' relates to speed. Athletes at all levels are constantly trying to improve their speed. Parents often ask me what they should do to help their children excel in sports like football, soccer and basketball? Well, if you get your children to run just 2 kilometres every morning and every evening, by the end of the week they will be 28 kilometres away! Jokes aside, there is no doubt that the single best thing you can do for young people after the age of 12 who want to do well in field sports is to train them for speed.

Speed training is not appropriate for everyone who leads an active lifestyle, though for those who need it, it's the number 1 priority. It can be done. You can get quicker!

Too often athletes are prematurely classified as being slow or 'one-paced' without any real analysis of their true physical characteristics. What you inherit from your parents in regard to physical make-up and natural inclination for speed is an important factor. However, while there is no doubt that bloodlines affect speed, the relative number of fast and slow twitch muscle fibres you are born with is not the sole determinant of your speed.

Fast twitch muscle fibres are those that contract quickly and powerfully and tire rapidly, sometimes within

5–6 seconds. The power athlete has a predominance of fast twitch fibres. He or she is explosively fast and powerful but may struggle to sustain that intensity of effort for any period of time. People with a predominance of fast twitch fibres are best suited to quick bursts of absolute effort with rest periods in between, so that these fast twitch fibres can recover and prepare for their next dynamic burst.

Slow twitch fibres can repeatedly contract for long periods without fatiguing greatly, but they can't generate anywhere near the force of the fast twitch type. Endurance type athletes may lack fast acceleration in running or any other movement, though they can keep performing for extended periods.

We're all born with some of each type. Muscle biopsies of sprinters have revealed ratios of up to 80% fast to 20% slow twitch fibres. You could expect Olympic 100-metre gold medallists to have this sort of genetic advantage for speed, while ultra marathoners can be as low as 30% fast twitch to 70% slow twitch. Most people are in the 50–70% of fast to slow twitch range.

The general scientific opinion is that you cannot change fast twitch into slow twitch fibres. You cannot reproduce or somehow grow new fast twitch fibres. Maximising speed is a matter of making the most of what you've got. Many people believe that because genetic make-up can't be altered, you can't learn to be faster. This school of thought is wrong because it completely ignores two vital factors: strength and technique.

The first sure way there is to improve your pace is to increase the strength of your hip flexors. The hip flexors are the muscles in your lower abdomen and at the front of your thighs. Their function is to lift your legs with each stride when you run. Strong hip flexors don't look as impressive as bulging biceps but they do provide the force for that 'pumping piston' high knee lift needed to accelerate quickly off the mark when sprinting. Well-developed hip flexors are not immediately obvious to the eye though they can help generate great speed within a couple of metres of take-off.

You will develop strong hip flexors through specific sit up type exercises, high knee running drills and leg lifts on a hip flexor machine. It's a matter of progressively overloading these muscles so that they become more powerful and therefore faster. If your legs are moving faster, you'll run faster.

The second way to improve speed is through technique. To understand the importance of technique, compare the running styles of sprinter Michael Jonson and basketballer Andrew Gaze. Michael keeps his head still, his arms pumping forward in a smooth and controlled manner, his shoulders square and his knee lift high. Andrew tends to roll his arms across his body, and carries his knees low, with his feet moving out and around rather than straight through. The result is a bobbing head and a struggling, lunging gait. Andrew uses a lot more energy and takes a lot more time to get from point A to point B. Regardless of the number of fast or slow twitch fibres you have and the strength of your hip flexors, technique counts. Any athlete from age 12 onwards will benefit from concentrating on, and periodically reminding themselves of, the basics of correct technique. All young people would be well advised to have their technique analysed and corrected so that the proper habits become ingrained as they grow.

The main points of technique are to keep your head still and shoulders slightly forward. This promotes balance. The arms swing through with a constant elbow bend of almost 90 degrees. The arms shouldn't open and close as you run, they stay bent and push through and forward from the shoulders. You can practise this in front of a mirror to make sure your arms aren't pushing across your body and therefore wasting energy and upsetting your balance.

Legwork starts with strong hip flexors and a conscious high knee lift. At take off, try to take more quick steps rather than longer strides. This is the basis of acceleration. There are dozens of sportspeople, even at senior levels, who think that they can't improve their speed because they're stuck with what they were born with. If only they knew that it's not genetics holding them back, but a lack of functional strength and proper technique. It's really a simple formula. You need an efficient technique and functional strength to develop speed in any movement. If you have these, then you will maximise the use of the fast twitch fibres you do have. Who knows how many fast twitch fibres you have that aren't being used to their optimum? They may just be waiting for a chance to use their power and boost your career. When it comes to sport, speed saves.

WATERWORLD

You can never have too many workout options. Your program should include some cross-training substitutes and low-impact alternatives to provide the mental and physical variety you need to stay fit, focused and injury free. Swimming fills all these needs. It's totally different from any other form of exercise and it's the ultimate in low-impact exercise. In effect it's no impact.

To achieve a training effect, you must elevate your heart rate into your training zone. You must also maintain this level for a period of at least 15 minutes to score

1 exercise point. At least 30 minutes is preferable to score 2 points and make your trip to the pool worthwhile.

If you aren't an experienced swimmer, you are unlikely to feel comfortable swimming continuously for longer than 15 minutes unless the word crawl describes your speed as well as your stroke. It's the classic catch 22. If you swim too slowly, you don't elevate your heart rate into your training zone, and if you swim faster, you can't keep the speed up for long enough to score exercise points. For these reasons, the swimming workouts have been designed to guarantee that you score exercise points. The workouts begin with continuous swims of only 500 metres, followed by 'intervals' of shorter distances at faster speeds with rest periods in between each effort. It's the same concept as circuit training.

Interval swimming does not require good stroke technique, because it relies on intensity and recovery rather than skill level. Interval swimming virtually assures you of a worthwhile workout because the fast tempos elevate your heart rate into the appropriate range. The rest periods between intervals allow your heart rate to recover when it has exceeded the high side of your training zone and even though interval swimming is more intense than continuous low tempo swimming, it is still one of the least injurious workouts you can choose.

You will be the best judge of where to start on the 12 levels that follow. If you're undecided on a choice between two levels, start on the lower of the two. It's much easier to adjust upward than it is to adjust downward. The training time has been deliberately set at around 45 minutes per session so that each workout will be worth 3 exercise points.

Level 1 should take around 14 minutes for the 500-metre swim followed by a 4-minute rest, 50 seconds for each 50-metre dash and 90 seconds for each recovery between swims. Level 12 will require just over 22 minutes for the continuous swim, 3 minutes for rest and just over 20 minutes for the intervals.

Level 1	500 metres continuous
	4 min rest
	10 x 50 metre swims at fast tempo with 90 sec rest
Level 2	500 metres continuous
	4 min rest
	10 x 50 metre swims at fast tempo with 75 sec rest
Level 3	600 metres continuous
	4 min rest
	10 x 50 metre swims at fast tempo with 60 sec rest
Level 4	750 metres continuous
	4 min rest
	12 x 50 metre swims at fast tempo with 75 sec rest
Level 5	750 metres continuous
	3 min rest
	12 x 50 metre swims at fast tempo with 60 sec rest
Level 6	1000 metres continuous
	3 min rest
	10 x 50 metre swims at fast tempo with 90 sec rest
Level 7	1000 metres continuous
	3 min rest
	10 x 50 metre swims at fast tempo with 75 sec rest
Level 8	1000 metres continuous
	3 min rest
	10 x 50 metre swims at fast tempo with 60 sec rest
Level 9	1250 metres continuous
	3 min rest
	10 x 50 metre swims at fast tempo with 75 sec rest
Level 10	1250 metres continuous
	3 min rest

	10 x 50 metre swims at fast tempo with 60 sec rest
Level 11	1500 metres continuous
	3 min rest
	10 x 50 metre swims at fast tempo with 75 sec rest
Level 12	1500 metres continuous
	3 min rest
	12 x 50 metre swims at fast tempo with 60 sec rest

HOT SPOTS

Tummy, hips and thighs are still the hot spots. These are the areas we'd all like to see a little leaner and a lot flatter. The best way to shed unwanted kilograms around your middle is to exercise in a manner that will burn calories for 60 minutes, 4 times each week. If you are scoring your 4 exercise points on each exercise day, you will be doing well.

You can 'go the extra mile' by doing hundreds of sit ups to tone your stomach muscles, but the sit ups won't work without the regular kilojoules burning. There is no such thing as spot reduction.

Strong abdominals are more than visually appealing; they perform the primary function of flexing the trunk forward. Every time we bend over or stand up we need our abdominals working for us. Strong abdominals are also the most effective back protection you will ever have.

The best abdominal exercise is the crunch. The crunch can be performed with an 'ab trainer' machine or by lying on your back with your knees bent and your feet resting on a chair. Do not straighten your legs as this forces the body into a V position which creates extreme pressure through your lower back. As well as being uncomfortable, this does nothing to strengthen or tone your muscles, so remember to keep your knees bent. Before you start, push your buttocks as close in toward the chair as possible so that both your knees and hips are bent to a 90-degree angle. This stops the psoas muscle at the top of your thigh from doing too much of the work. After all, we want the abdominals to be the prime movers and greatest beneficiaries from the exercise.

The positioning of your hands depends on your level of conditioning. If you are a beginner, rest your hands on top of your thighs and slide them toward your knees as your body raises upward. The intermediate position is to grasp your ear lobe between thumb and forefinger of each hand while your elbows point outwards. This prevents you from pulling on your neck. This is definitely something to avoid. The advanced position is to cross your arms behind your head so that each hand rests against the opposite shoulder blade throughout the exercise. Whichever hand position you use, it's vital that your shoulders leave the floor before your lower back, because it is this movement that is controlled by the stomach. If you arch your back, you'll achieve nothing but problems. If you're feeling pressure in your neck, your legs or lower back, then your technique needs more work. You should be feeling pressure in the abdominals and you will when you get your technique right.

Start with 4 sets of 12 crunches with a minute's rest between sets. Aim to be able to do 4 sets of 25 within 3 weeks of commencing an abdominal program. You can do this exercise daily, and I hope you will. It will take you 15 minutes to complete these 4 sets and you will earn 1 exercise point each time.

The crunch itself will not be enough. Once you're up to 4 sets of 25 standard crunches, add a variation. Keep doing your crunches and add another 4 sets of 12, this time performing the crunch with alternate twists to the left and right knee. These rotations place more emphasis on your transverse abdominals, which run across your abdomen and give you the washboard look. By the end of the sixth week you should be doing a total of 8 sets of 25: half straight-up crunches and half that should be crunches with a twist. It may sound more like a drink order than an exercise program; however, if you keep to the 8 sets and gradually increase your reps toward your ultimate aim of 50 each time, you'll eventually be doing a total of 400 crunches each day!

You'll also need to keep working on stamina and burning calories. This will come from walking, riding, swimming or any other continuous moderate exercise you do 4 times during the week to score the other exercise points you need.

ROW AT HOME

What's the best form of home exercise? It's a common question and without doubt, the answer is rowing. If you want an aerobic activity that trains the abdominals at the same time as your heart and lungs, then you should row! Enthusiasts will want to be on the water, but you can achieve the same benefit in the gym or at home using a rowing machine.

Rowing provides a cardiovascular burn along with both upper and lower body strength and conditioning. To row correctly you should start each stroke with your arms straight and your legs bent. You start the 'pull' with your legs and then quickly add the arm component. Each stroke ends with the legs fully extended and the arms fully bent. As you slide forward in the recovery phase, reach as far forward as you can. This will maximise the power of your pull and the length of your next stroke.

In your first session you may feel uncoordinated and tight in the gluteal muscles of your rear end. During the second session you should start to develop some rhythm and by the third you should be rowing smoothly.

If you are new to rowing set the resistance or the level of difficulty on the machine very conservatively. Work on your technique and try to achieve a 10-minute session on your first attempt. Once you get used to your machine, you may find yourself enjoying or enduring a fully self-contained 45–60 minute session (3–4 exercise points) without feeling the need or having the energy to do anything else when you finish.

Because rowing machines are so different, your best guide to exercise efficiency is your own pulse rate. Once again a heart-rate monitor will prove invaluable. Try to keep within 5 beats of your heart-rate target. Keep to a steady rate of 20 to 22 long, fluent strokes per minute. Only increase your tempo up toward 24 to 28 strokes per minute when you are sure your heart rate won't exceed your training zone target. If you find yourself rowing any faster than this, make sure you are still reaching well forward and pulling right back with each stroke. If you do this, you will make sure your abdominals are really contributing to the effort each time your upper body bends forward and pulls into the rowing stroke.

If rowing isn't an option, but you'd like to target your buttocks while burning calories at the same time, you just can't beat stair climbing, especially if you take them 2 at a time. Our gluteal muscles are the prime movers when we take long uphill steps; so give these muscles a toning workout at the same time you're burning some calories. It's best to start by climbing and descending 1 flight of steps at a time. When you're ready, it's a great workout to climb 1, descend 1, climb 2, descend 1, climb 3, descend 1, climb 4, descend 1, then finally climb 5 and descend 5. Rest for 30 seconds then start all over again. Repeat the entire routine another 3 times for a terrific workout. For safety reasons, on the way down you should make foot contact with every step. Don't start leaping 3 or more steps at a time when you are out of breath and trying to recover. Recovery is a part of the program. Take your time on the way down and do the hard work on the way up.

STAYING SANE WHEN INJURED

The final fitness comment relates to the dreaded times when you find you've injured yourself. I hope you will avoid injury by following the Every Day Counts system. If you do sustain an injury, try to keep things in perspective.

One of the main reasons we train relates to self-esteem. We want to feel good about ourselves, and being fit promotes a positive self-image. Active people have a positive aura. Others pick up on this and they will want to be around you. The problem is that when we're injured, our self-esteem can become dented. We don't like having something wrong with us; it just doesn't feel natural to rest and be inactive, and who wants to give up the fitness and performance levels they have achieved through a lot of hard work?

The temptation to return to your program will be strong. Physically and emotionally, you will want to be back out there and so, it you're not careful, you skimp on the rehab work and return to full training too quickly. The theme is all too common. The key words are frustration and impatience. The answer is to be calm and patient.

Regardless of how much treatment you have, how much cross training you do, how many nutritional supplements you take and how much mental rehearsal you perform, your body will need rest. There's a good chance that lack of rest may have been the reason you developed the injury in the first place!

If you are considering surgery as a means of fixing the problem, think hard. When it comes to comparing surgical scars, an increasing number of people can join in the conversation. Many people are now being operated on for injuries and ailments that were previously treated with rest and rehabilitation. Undoubtedly, surgical techniques have been at the forefront in the advancement of sports medicine over the past decade. The most common operations are for joint damage, stress fractures, hernia and soft tissue detachments.

Even though many complaints are now surgically repaired in an advanced manner, it must be remembered that surgery is not a cure all. Complete recovery after surgery is not guaranteed. However, if you are unfortunate enough to rupture the anterior cruciate ligament in your knee, then surgery is the right option. The ligament will not reconnect naturally and an operation is the logical choice to prevent you from having a painful and unstable knee for the rest of your life. On the other hand, ligament strains may only be partial and, in time, with specialist exercise and therapy the strain may knit and heal itself. This is just one example. Many conditions falling into the 'operative' category are marginal and may respond quickly and well to rest and thorough rehabilitation. They may call them 'minor operations,' the definition of which is an operation performed on someone else!

Stress fractures often respond better to rest than surgical pinning and many people who undergo groin or other inguinal operations report that even after long and arduous post-operative rehabilitation, the original pain remains or returns as soon as activity is resumed.

The final decision is yours and no one else's. Certainly take advice from and respect the opinions of orthopaedic surgeons, but remember that as surgeons, their professional expertise revolves around a commitment to the precise science of surgery. They may be so convinced that theirs is the best way to help you that they become subconsciously biased against the less intrusive alternatives.

Never underestimate the natural healing power of the human body. We are a unique organism. There are many successful instances of people who've opted against exposing their joints to surgery and the associated problems of general anaesthesia, of oxygen entering a joint, the potential for future arthritis and the possibility of less than certain success in the operation.

What do I do now?

1 Keep being aware of the fat content, in grams, of the food you eat during the course of each day for the remainder of your 14-day trial.

2 Keep scoring your exercise in terms of 1 point for every 15 minutes spent when you are active more than you are resting.

3 Score your 'training to keep fit' exercise in exactly the same manner. That's 1 point for every 15 minutes spent training to improve your fitness.

4 Read the final chapter, The Extra Edge, and be ready for the real challenge to begin.

11

THE EXTRA EDGE

*'You win some, you lose some. Only mediocre
people are always at their best.'*

W Somerset Maugham

EASY STEPS TO A BETTER BODY

Strong convictions precede great actions. As you begin
your 9-month challenge, you need to reaffirm some of the
basics. These basics will reinforce the thoughts you should
now be thinking and the actions you should now be
taking. Please refer back to this section from time to time
to check your mental attitude and progress.

1 You don't have to be perfect! Not everyone has the
   commitment to treat their body like a temple, but
   most of us have a real desire to look and feel strong
   and healthy. The basic things you do every day will
   shape your body, manage your stress and control
   your eating.
2 Muscles are like plasticine. They are brittle and
   inflexible when cold but pliable and easily stretched
   when warm. Warming up assists performance and
   prevents injury.

3 Once you've established the habit, morning is a great time to exercise. Lots of people hate the idea of working out in the morning, but it's the only time most people don't have other priorities or responsibilities in their lives. Our plan isn't to skimp on work, family or social time. Our plan is to incorporate them.

4 Don't dwell on the hours of sleep you're losing, but focus on the hours you're investing in yourself and the rewards it will bring. You have to invest some energy to get a lot more back in return.

5 Having said all of this, some people still cannot stand the idea of training in the mornings. If you are exercising at other times during the day, record exercise appointments in your diary. If you must make a change, treat your workout with the same respect you would give any other appointment. Schedule an alternative time to train right away.

6 Find a good training partner, someone who can become your conscience, coach and safety spotter all in one. When geese fly in formation, the whole flock adds 71% greater flying range compared with each bird flying on its own. As each bird flaps its wings, it creates an uplift for the bird immediately following. Humans also work well together. It's much easier to let yourself down by not turning up than it is to let someone else down.

7 When you reach a food, exercise and pressure target, reward yourself. Don't just let your achievement slip past. When you set yourself a target and pay the price to reach that target, you've earned the reward. Take it! Start by making yourself take your 7 daily rewards when you reach your points targets.

8 Food is our fuel and we truly are what we eat. All our tissues are being continually regenerated and replaced, even our muscles and bones. It's called the aging process. Healthy eating controls and delays the aging process.

9 It's not just lack of knowledge that stops us from eating good foods; it's lack of will. We have to find a way to stop gorging ourselves with fat. The key is to limit your intake to between 40 and 50 grams per day.

10 Hard body foods include grain breads, dry baked or boiled potatoes, all fruits and most vegetables, low-fat dairy products, unrefined pasta and rice, beans, lean meat, fish and chicken, fruit juice and egg whites. These foods should be most of what you eat each day.

11 Soft body foods include cakes, biscuits, lollies, soft drink, alcohol (except your first two drinks each day), anything cooked in fat, most sauces and toppings, and too much tea or coffee. These foods should be less than one fifth of what you eat each day with the fat content being between 40 and 50 grams.

12 Alcohol is a drug, but it is very much toward the positive end of the drugs spectrum. It offers nutritional and therapeutic value when taken in moderation, but too much of a good thing causes problems. Your first 2 alcoholic drinks of the day are +1 food choices. After that, they are all negative. Try for at least 2 alcohol-free days a week just to give your liver a rest.

13 Don't fall for the propaganda that it's only red wine that may offer protection against heart disease. While the skin of the red grape houses some

beneficial antioxidants, it's the alcohol that offers the health benefit, not specifically only the alcohol found in red wine. Swallow the wine; don't swallow what the marketing campaign would have you believe. Keep monitoring your fat in grams.

14 Smoking is a definite no. Of the people who develop lung cancer, 97% are smokers. Smoking also hardens arteries, increases blood pressure, reduces lung capacity, diseases the liver, costs a ridiculous amount of cash and gives you bad breath. Smoking is like puckering up to an exhaust pipe. The same gases that come out the back of a car come out the butt of a cigarette.

15 Water is the hard body fluid. It has no calories, is non-toxic even in large doses, it dilutes poisons and flushes out wastes. If you are not drinking at least 1.5 litres of water daily, you're not trying hard enough.

16 Antioxidant vitamins are hard body supplements. They can protect our heart and immune systems and have been reliably researched now for 10 years. Vitamins A, C and E, that's the recipe. Recent publicity about potential vitamin side-effects applies only with massive dosages. Sensible supplements can add to your vitality and health protection.

17 Whatever type of exercise you do, breathe out with effort. Exhaling releases tension as you produce force, exhaling adds impetus to your movement and it encourages you to breathe in again. Never hold your breath when working out.

18 Take 5 minutes to warm down. It's asking too much of your body to go from 'full throttle to full stop' without a period of adjustment. Ease out of your work outs to reduce stress on your muscular

and nervous systems. Walking is a great way to warm down.

19 Tomorrow's another day; if not, it's all over. Tomorrow never comes. If you're having a frantic week or a chaotic month, don't delay working on your lifestyle until things settle down. Chances are you have a busy life and things won't be settling down for the next few decades unless *you* make them. Don't win at work and lose at life. Start now.

20 Breathe deeply every day. It eliminates wastes, strengthens muscles, reduces tension and helps keep the balance between your conscious and subconscious minds. It's the most natural health exercise of all.

21 Fight for quality time. It might be your exercise time. It might be your pressure time. It might be different time altogether. You now have the tools to deal with pressure in your life. You have to strive for quality time. It is one of your basic human needs. Don't be a martyr, look after yourself. Lack of quality time may have been one of the motivations for you to read and hopefully embrace Every Day Counts. Quality time is essential. Take some.

THE JOURNEY IS THE DESTINATION

A young man was standing beside a narrow, smooth flowing river gazing at the beautiful scene on the far bank. He was pondering life. His mind was consumed with competitive and material wants, his spirit was bogged down by a lack of meaning and he forced his body to cope with constant abuse and neglect.

The man's life was filled to overflowing. Demands were high and time was short. It seemed that there was always something that needed to be done. On the far bank of the river people were able to live one integrated life. It was as if on his side of the river, time controlled people, but on the far side, people controlled time. If only I could get across the river to the other side, thought the man. If only I could find a bridge.

He thought about it a little more, then realised that he already had everything he needed to construct a bridge. All the materials and the know-how were available; all he really needed was the time to make a start. Time was the one thing he didn't have.

The young man would have pondered some more, but his mind wanted action, his body wanted feeding and his spirit was looking for fulfillment. He decided he would return to the riverbank soon. He'd finalise his bridge design and make a start; he'd do it as soon as he had a chance, as soon as things settled down.

As the man matured, he grew in wealth and stature and was still as busy as ever. His physical being had begun to decline so he decided to postpone building his bridge until he had more time and felt better. Looking back at his younger days, he couldn't understand why he hadn't just swum across. It was only a short distance across the river and the current was mild. Even now part of him wanted to dive in and take the plunge.

Then he thought about his listless and painful body and knew the effort was now beyond him. It seemed so simple looking back. Why hadn't he done something earlier? Why hadn't he lived the way he wanted to live?

The years passed as if they were months as the man pandered to the competing demands of mind, body and spirit. Before he knew it he was prematurely old. The old man returned to the river to imagine the bridge he had never had time to build. As he gazed out across the river, he was struck by a blinding flash of the obvious —

remember the BFO? — and a harsh truth about life: the journey becomes the destination.

On his side of the river some people had strong bodies, some had powerful minds and others were consumed by the spiritual. Very few seemed able to get all three facets of life working together.

On the far side he could see that financially rich people didn't have to be emotionally bankrupt. He could see that successful, important people could still have time to do what they wanted. He could see men playing with their children and women secure in their own self-image rather than being slaves to other people's expectations of how they should look or act.

At last he could see what he was and what he wanted to be; it was just too late. As John Lennon sang when the man was still young, 'Life is what happens while you're busy making other plans.'

If you are lucky, your health is still intact. Don't neglect it. Opportunity is knocking right now, an opportunity to live in the Health Zone by making Every Day Count. It's an opportunity to live on the right side of the river.

MAKING A PACT

Crossing the bridge is a metaphor for changing your habits. None of us can go back and make a new beginning, but as the saying goes, we can start now and begin a new ending.

Most human behaviour is based on habits, and habits are hard to change. This is exactly why we need the Every Day Counts system.

Let's take one more look at food. There's no doubt that the easiest way to burn off the excess kilojoules found in a doughnut is not to eat the doughnut in the first place! Unfortunately, for most of us, eating lean on a day-in and day-out basis is much easier to say than it is to do. Congratulations if you are strong-willed enough to make this happen. The reality for most people is that we need help to control our urge for fatty food. It is a habit. Exercise and stress management are also habits. Once they are ingrained into your lifestyle they will be harder to give up than they were to start.

Every Day Counts will change your health habits. By now you will have tried out components of the system and tried it out for part of your 14-day trial period. When you complete this 14-day trial, it will be time to begin the program in earnest. It's now time to make a PACT with yourself. PACT is an acronym to help you change your health habits.

P stands for Planning. Plan a regular work-out schedule that will suit your lifestyle. Put your program on paper and include some detail so that your plan doesn't end up being just a 'verbal contract'. Make sure you are committing to 60 minutes on 4 out of every 7 days. Plan to reach your exercise points target of 4 points on the 4 exercise days each week. Plan to reach your daily food target of 12 points and plan to reach your daily pressure target of 4 points.

A stands for Action. This is when you try out your planned program. It's exactly what you are doing right now. Use what's left of your 14-day trial to see what works for you. Be prepared to modify your eating plans during this action phase. You should also settle on the right number of eating choices, remembering that 25 food choices is standard with a higher option of 30 choices and a lower option of 20 choices. Please try to keep within this range.

You should be finding out the most convenient training times, the best locations and duration for your exercise sessions. Decide whether you are going to walk, jog, run, swim, box, and work with weights, ride, blade or slide. By the end of this 'action time' you should have a firm idea of exactly what exercise and what time segments (15 minutes, 30 minutes, 45 minutes or 60 minutes) work best for you.

Here's an example of a weekly schedule that will get you moving, and earn you 4 exercise points on the 4 exercise days.

Monday	5-km walk or run (40 min), stretch (5 min) and 15-min body weight circuit. Total 60 min = 4 points
Tuesday	Rest
Wednesday	Swim session: 1 km swim (30 min) followed by 10 x 50 m faster swims with 60 sec recovery between each (30 min). Total 60 min = 4 points
Thursday	Rest
Friday	3-km warm up run or walk (20 min), 5 x 200 m easy paced run or walk throughs with 60 sec recoveries (15 min), 3 km warm down and stretch (25 min). Total 60 min = 4 points
Saturday	Rest
Sunday	25 km road cycle (40 min), body weight exercise circuit (15 min) and stretch (5 min). Total 60 min = 4 points

During this action phase you should also be fine-tuning your pressure blockers and coping techniques. Experiment with your stress management techniques to work out the best ways for you to manage stress and earn your daily pressure points. The action phase is vital because lots of people make the mistake of making a premature commitment. They go straight from the planning phase to the commitment phase without having ever tried out their plans in the real world. It is vital for you to put your plans into practice before drawing a line in the sand and saying to yourself, I will not retreat!

Right now you are probably somewhere right in the middle of your action phase. When your 14-day trial is over, so too will be your action phase.

You're now half way toward making your PACT. The next pitfall people face is to get this far on a new plan, and then fail because they're not really committed to their cause. Everyone plans and some people act. *You* can set yourself apart by making a commitment.

C stands for Commitment. This is decision time! You've made your plans and had an opportunity to adjust and modify them in the 'Action' phase. Your plans are realistic. The Every Day Counts standards have already helped hundreds of people. We know it works and it can work for you.

If you make yourself a commitment now, there's no going back. Right now, I am asking you for a *Yes*, a firm commitment to incorporate the Every Day Counts system for the next 9 months of your life.

You are about to draw that line in the sand, and once you do, there's no crossing back over. Don't insult yourself by paying lip service to a commitment if you're not really serious. This is crunch time. As the old saying goes, 'If you don't stand for something, you'll fall for anything.' It's a big commitment but one I can promise you will be worthwhile.

Seek the support of someone you can trust. You can't fly like an eagle if you're surrounding yourself with turkeys. Please confirm your commitments to yourself now and write them on the following page.

My Commitments

Every Day Counts

Food: I commit to earning _____ points each day. I will have _____ food choices each day.

Exercise: I commit to earning _____ points on four days each week.

Stress Management: I commit to earning _____ pressure points each day.

Other commitments I wish to make:

_____

_____

_____

_____

_____

_____

_____

_____

_____

_____

_____

_____

_____

_____

T stands for Test. Sooner or later you are going to be tested. You may not see it coming, but it will arrive. I guarantee it!

Your test might be the shrill sound of the alarm on a cold, wet morning when you had planned to go for a 60-minute walk. It might be a taste temptation when you've already had enough negative food points on that day and you've already used up your humanity day for that week. It might even be just a small voice telling you that your weight is under control, your legs are sore and it would be easier just to go back to the way you were. Your test may even be that critical moment that you either allow yourself to get angry or decide to keep yourself calm.

You may not even know you've been tested until the moment has come and gone. In reality, you'll face many tests over the next 9 months. While the ultimate goal is worth the sacrifices you will be making, each test you pass along the way will be a victory in itself. Every time you choose the apple instead of the cake, each time you choose to exercise instead of being sedentary and each time you choose not to get angry will make you stronger and move you closer to a fantastic way of life.

Make your PACT: Plan, Act, Commit and be Tested. It's not just the final achievement you'll enjoy; it's all the benefits along the way. It's the crossing of the bridge, not just the magic place on the other side. The journey becomes the destination.

A FINAL WORD

Thanks for making it this far. If you've made the decision to give the program a go, the hardest part is already behind you. Once you make a decision, all of the doubts tend to fall away. You'll find it a relief to get started.

Getting out of bed for an early morning workout is enormously difficult if you go to sleep kidding yourself that you'll see how you feel when the alarm goes off. It's much easier when you have already made your mind up the night before. It's much easier when there is no decision to make. That's the way it has to be when you're making Every Day Count.

If you are still unsure about trying the program, experiment with it until you make a firm decision either way. Don't 'start the climb until it's time'.

I'd like to leave you with two thoughts. The first is a saying from a great friend of mine, Mark (Muddy) Waters. As Australia's leading tennis conditioning expert, Mark has seen the world 10 times or more and worked closely with just as many champion players. He's picked up a lot of wisdom along the way. Mark's favourite saying about life is simply, 'The things we regret are the things that we don't do.' I think he's right.

Finally, there is a very powerful quote about overcoming adversity. It says, 'If you should achieve any kind of success and develop superior qualities in life, chances are it will be because of the manner in which you meet the defeat that will come to you, just as it will come to all.'

We all face problems and challenges in our lives. We can't conquer them all at the first attempt, but when at last we do, the taste of success is so much sweeter.

This is one battle you can win. Live the life you want.

What do I do now?

1 Make a firm commitment to make Every Day Count for the next 9 months.
2 Score your 12 food points each day.
3 Score your 4 exercise points on 4 days each week.
4 Score your 4 pressure points each day.
5 Use your humanity day each week when you need it.

THE LAST PAGE

The Every Day Counts system is designed to become redundant after 9 months.

The concept of Every Day Counts is to use a system to help you bridge the gap between healthy lifestyle desires and healthy lifestyle actions. Do not use the system forever.

Use the system to construct your own bridge. Get to the other side of the river. Once you have achieved long-term healthy life practices, there will still be one more challenge for you to face.

Enjoy it!

Appreciate and value the life you've worked to achieve. Enjoy the energy and vitality that comes from healthy eating, regular exercise and managing pressure. Be secure in your long-term health. Take satisfaction from being in control of your destiny rather than a victim of circumstance.

What a great way to live. Above all else, remember this: You can't start living the good life until you stop wishing for a better one.

Appendix 1: Fast track

The next few pages summarise the Every Day Counts system. You can use this guide as a ready reference for how the system operates and how you can incorporate it into your daily life.

POINTS TARGETS
FOR FOOD, EXERCISE AND PRESSURE

Food points target	— 12 points each day
Exercise points target	— 4 points per day on 4 days per week
	— There are 3 rest days each week
	— No exercise points are needed on rest days
Pressure points target	— 4 points each day

TOTAL POINTS TARGETS

On each of the 4 exercise days your total target is:
12 food points + 4 exercise points + 4 pressure points
= 20 points

On each of the 3 non-exercise days your total target is:
12 food points + 4 pressure points = 16 points

EARNING POINTS

FOOD

- Every food choice you make is rated as +1, 0 or −1 point.
- You can make up to a total of 25 food choices each day.

- A food choice is defined as being any food or drink that weighs up to 200 grams. A food or drink choice weighing more than 200 grams counts as 2 food choices.
- From those 25 choices, your daily food challenge is to achieve a net score of 12 points. An example would be 16 × '+1' food or drink choices, 4 × '−1' choices, and 4 × '0' choices (16 − 4 + 0 = 12 points).
- You can earn up to 2 additional food points (e.g. 16 x '+1' choices, 2 × '−1' choices and 7 × '0' choices = 14 points) on any day to make up for a points shortage in exercise or pressure points. Your maximum possible food score is limited to 14 points. Even if you somehow managed to eat 25 x '+1' choices, your food score for that day would still be 14 points.
- You may use these 2 additional food points to make up for a shortfall in the exercise or pressure areas, in order to reach your overall daily target.
- Your recommended maximum fat intake each day is between 40 and 50 grams.
- The system is identical for both sexes.

Options

- People who are 'big eaters' and weigh in excess of 90 kilograms may opt to have 30 daily food choices instead of 25 choices. If you take this option you will have a daily food target of 15 points rather than the standard 12 points.
- People weighing less than 55 kilograms may opt to have only 20 food choices instead of 25 choices each day. If you take this option you will have a daily food target of 10 points rather than the standard 12 points.
- A full listing and rating of foods is contained in Appendix 2.

EXERCISE

- Award yourself 1 point for 15 minutes of continual activity.
- All exercise rates the same, regardless of intensity.
- Any activity that is continuous and requires you to be active more than you are passive qualifies as exercise. Time is the critical factor rather than intensity.
- Your target is 4 exercise points (1 hour of exercise) on 4 days each week.
- You may earn 2 additional points by exercising for an extra 30 minutes on any or all of your 4 exercise days each week.
- You may use these 2 additional exercise points to make up for a shortfall in the food or pressure areas, in order to reach your overall daily target.
- You cannot earn exercise points during the 3 rest days each week.
- Exercise points have been explained in detail in Chapter 4.

PRESSURE

- Pressure points are scored on the basis of 1 point for every 5 minutes you invest in managing pressure and controlling stress in your life.
- Your target is 4 pressure points (20 minutes) each day.
- Activities that enable you to deal with pressure qualify for pressure points. Examples are deep breathing, relaxation, spa and massage.
- You may earn 2 additional pressure points by countering stress for an extra 10 minutes on any day.

- You may use these 2 additional pressure points to make up for a shortfall in the food or exercise areas, in order to reach your overall daily target.
- Pressure points have been explained in detail in Chapters 7 and 8.

REWARDS

Rewards are an integral part of the system and must be established prior to beginning the program.

- A reward is earned each day for the first 7 days when your daily points targets are met.
- A reward is then earned each week for the next 7 weeks when your daily points targets are met on at least 6 out of the 7 days in that week.
- A reward is then earned each month for 7 months when your daily points targets are met on no less than 6 days out of each week during that month.
- You set you own rewards (see Chapter 2).

HUMANITY DAYS

- There is 1 day in every 7 when you are not required to reach your target. This is your humanity day.
- You can fall short of your food, exercise, pressure or total target during a humanity day without breaking the system or losing your designated reward. Humanity days are not an excuse to binge and over-indulge. They are designed to allow for our human frailties. They recognise that there may be 1 day each week when we don't quite reach our target. Humanity days allow you to miss 1 day's target without breaking the system (see more about humanity days in Chapter 2).

Appendix 2: Food lists

FOOD LISTS BY GROUP

Food Type	Rating	Comments	Fat in grams (100 grams unless specified otherwise)
Fruit			
Apples	+1		<1
Apricots	+1		<1
Avocados	−1	Good choice if you need some fat in your diet and want to avoid cholesterol; cholesterol free but still high in fat	20
Bananas	+1		<1
Blackberries	+1		<1
Blackcurrants	+1		<1
Cherries	+1		<1
Coconut	−1	Fresh	27
"	−1	Dessicated	62
Currants	+1		<1
Dates	+1		<1
Figs	+1		<1
Fruit salad	+1		<1
Grapefruit	+1		<1
Grapes	+1		<1
Guava	+1		<1
Kiwi fruit	+1		<1
Lemons	+1		<1
Lychees	+1		<1
Mandarins	+1		<1
Mangoes	+1		<1
Melon	+1		<1
Nectarines	+1		<1

Oranges	+1		<1
Passionfruit	+1		<1
Paw-paw	+1		<1
Peaches	+1		<1
Pears	+1		<1
Pineapple	+1		<1
Plums	+1		<1
Prunes	+1		<1
Raisins	+1		<1
Raspberries	+1		<1
Rhubarb	+1		<1
Strawberries	+1		<1
Sultanas	+1		<1
Tangerines	+1		<1

Vegetables

Asparagus	+1		<1
Bamboo shoots	+1		<1
Beans	+1		<1
Beetroot	+1		<1
Broccoli	+1		<1
Brussel sprouts	+1		<1
Cabbage	+1		<1
Carrots	+1		<1
Cauliflower	+1		<1
Celery	+1		<1
Chick peas	+1		2
Chicory	+1		<1
Cucumber	+1		<1
Eggplant	+1		2
Fennel	+1		<1
Garlic	+1		<1
Gherkins	+1		<1
Ginger	+1		<1

Leeks	+1		<1
Lentils	+1		<1
Lettuce	+1		<1
Mushrooms	+1		<1
Olives	+1		2
Onions	+1		<1
Parsnip	+1		<1
Peas	+1		<1
Peppers	+1		<1
Potatoes	+1		<1
"	+1	Dry-baked in jackets	0
"	−1	Fried in oil; thick cut (>1cm thick)	14
"	−1	Roasted in oil	5
"	0	Mashed with butter or margerine	8
Pumpkin	+1		<1
"	−1	Roasted in oil	6
Radish	+1		<1
Soy beans	+1	Cooked	6
Spinach	+1		<1
Spring onions	+1		<1
Sweetcorn	+1		<1
Tofu	0		8
"	−1	Fried	16
Tomatoes	+1		<1
Zucchini	+1		<1

Breads

Bagel	+1		4 per bagel
Croissant	−1	The pastry high in fat	16
Crumpets	+1		2 per slice
Dark rye	+1		1 per slice
Focaccia	−1		7
Garlic bread	−1	Use of butter creates high fat content	18
Light rye	+1		1 per slice

Muffins	+1	Per small muffin	3 per slice
Multi-grain	+1		1 per slice
Naan	−1	High in fat, but good source of fibre	7 per serve
Pitta	+1		2
Raisin bread	+1		1 per slice
Sourdough	+1		1 per slice
Soy and linseed	+1		3 per slice
White	+1		1 per slice
White, fibre-increased	+1		2 per slice .
Wholemeal	+1	Almost 3 times richer in fibre than white bread	2 per slice

Cereals

All Bran	+1		2
Coco Pops	0	Contain more sugar than most cereals	<1
Cornflakes	+1		1
Crunchy Nut Corn Flakes	0		4
Just Right	+1		1
Muesli	−1	Toasted, high in fat	25
"	+1	Natural	5
Oat Bran	+1		3
Sultana Bran	+1		1
Special K	+1		1
Weetbix	+1		2
Porridge	+1		5
Rice Bubbles	+1		<1
Sustain	+1		3

Pastas

Pasta itself has little or no fat. It is the accompanying sauces that contribute all the fat. Any cream-based sauces are high in fat, therefore it is best to choose tomato-based sauces such as Napolitana.

Cannelloni	+1		1
Carbonara	−1		12
Fettucini	+1		<1
Gnocchi	+1	Potato gnocchi with cheese	1
Lasagna	0	With meat	6
"	+1	With vegetables	4
Macaroni	−1	Baked with cheese	13
"	+1	Wholewheat, no cheese	2
Ravioli	0	Meat filled	5
"	+1	Spinach and ricotta	3
Risotto	+1		4
Spaghetti	+1	Plain	<1
"	+1	Wholewheat	<1
Spaghetti bolognese		With oil	15
Tortellini	0		8

Crackers, grains and flours

Crispbread	0		5
Ricecakes	+1		<1
Taco shells	0		4
Water biscuits	0	Fat content varies; read label	
Arrowroot flour	+1		0
Barley	+1		2
Buckwheat flour	+1		2
Cornflour	+1		<1
Oat meal	+1		7
Rice	+1	Brown, boiled or steamed	1
"	−1	Brown, fried	7
"	+1	White, boiled or steamed	<1
"	−1	White, fried	6
Rye flour	+1		3
Semolina	+1		1
Soybean flour	−1	Full fat	17

"	+1	Low fat	1
Wheatgerm	+1		6
Wholewheat flour	+1		2
Wild rice	+1		3

Nuts and seeds

Nuts are generally quite high in fat, however, low in cholesterol. They are a poor choice if your aim is to lower your total fat intake.

Almonds	−1		55
Brazil nuts	0	Thought to reduce prostate cancer risk; balances high fat content	65
Cashew nuts	−1	Salted	45
Chestnuts	0		3
Hazelnuts	−1		61
Macadamia	−1		76
Peanuts	−1	Roasted, unsalted	49
"	−1	Roasted, salted	49
Pecan nuts	−1		71
Pine nuts	−1		51
Pistachio nuts	−1	Shelled	48
"	−1	Unshelled	28
Sesame seeds	−1		50
Sunflower seeds	−1		50
Walnuts	0	Help protect against heart disease	52

Legumes and beans

Alfalfa sprouts	+1		0
Baked beans	+1		<1
Black-eyed beans	+1		1
Broad beans	+1		<1
Cannellini beans	+1		<1
Chick peas	+1		2
Falafel	+1		8

Green beans	+1		<1
Haricot beans	+1		1
Kidney beans	+1		<1
Lentils	+1		<1
Lima beans	+1		<1
Mung beans	+1		<1
Peas	+1		<1
Pinto beans	+1		2
Soya beans	+1		6

Meats and poultry

It is important to note that even lean meats have moderate fat content and therefore consuming more than 200 grams can result in unacceptably high fat content. The fat content of meat and poultry will vary significantly depending on the cut and method of preparation.

Bacon	−1		35
Beef			
Mince	−1		10
"	+1	Extra lean	6
Meat pie	−1	At least 20 grams of fat per pie	20+
Silverside	−1		15
Bolognese sauce	−1		20
"	+1	No oil, lean meat	8
Chicken			
Breast	−1	With skin (animal skin high in saturated fats)	12
"	+1	Skinless, grilled	4
Fried	−1	17	
Barbecued	−1	With skin	13
"	+1	Skinless	8
Parmigiana	−1	Made with ham and cheese; increases fat content	22
Duck	0	Roast, skinless	10
"	−1	Roast, with skin	29
Frankfurters	−1		13

Ham	0	Can be high in fat	5
Hamburgers	−1	Home-made with lean meat, salad, no butter = +1	10
Heart, kidney, liver	0	Not fried	16
Hot dog	−1	High in fat, preservatives	15
Lamb chops	−1		31
"	0	Grilled, lean	12
Pork, new fashioned	+1		9
Salami	−1	High in fat	45
Sausage roll	−1		18
Sausages	−1		13
Steak			
Sirloin	−1		12
"	+1	Lean, trimmed and grilled	8
Porterhouse	−1	Tends to have high fat content	15
"	+1	Small, grilled, lean, trimmed	8
Rump	−1	Tends to have high fat content	15
"	+1	Small, grilled, lean, trimmed	5
T-bone	−1	Tends to have high fat content	12
Strassburg	−1		24
Turkey	+1		3
Veal	+1	Lean, grilled	4
Veal parmigiana	−1	Made with ham, cheese; increases fat content	20

Fish/Seafood

Most fish is quite low in fat, but again the method of cooking is vital. Any seafood fried in batter constitutes a score of −1.

Anchovies	−1	High in fat	14
Barramundi	+1		<1
Caviar	0		8
Cod	+1		<1
Crab	+1		1

Crayfish	+1		1
Fish and chips	−1	High in fat	25
Fish fingers	−1	Pre-fried, high in preservatives	16
Flake	+1		1
Flathead	+1		1
Flounder	+1		<1
Garlic prawns	−1		9
Haddock	+1		1
Herring	−1	High in fat	14
Lobster	+1		1
Mackerel	0		10
Mussel	0		2
Octopus (calamari)	+1	If fried score is −1	1
Oyster	0		1
Pilchards	+1	Steamed	3
Prawns	+1		2
Salmon	+1	No oil	5
Sardine	−1	Canned in oil, not drained	28
"	−1	Cannned in oil, drained	14
Scallop	+1		1
Snapper	+1		1
Trout	+1		3
Tuna	+1	Brine, water	3
"	−1	Canned in oil	22
Whiting	+1		1

Dairy products

Butter	−1		82
Margarine	−1		80

Cheese: most yellow cheeses are around 30 grams fat per 100 grams of weight.

Brie	−1		30
Camembert	−1		28

Cheddar	−1		38
Cottage	+1	Low in fat	14
Feta	−1		30
Mozzarella	−1		30
Parmesan	−1		28
Ricotta	+1	Low in fat	12
Swiss	−1		30
Cream	−1		35
Cream, sour	−1		18
Eggs	*	First two for the week count as +1, then −1	11
Fried	−1		18
Scrambled	−1		14
Ice cream	−1		24
Columbo	+1	Low fat variety of ice cream	8
Vitari	0		10
Milk			
Skim	+1		0
Rev or Physical	0		20
Whole	−1		40
Soy	0	Still relatively high in fat	16
Yoghurt			
Low-fat	+1		6
Regular	0		16

Snacks: sweet and savoury

Boiled sweets	0		0
Burger rings	−1		26
Carob cookies	−1	High in fat	25
Cheese and bacon balls	−1		34
Cheezles	−1		30
Chocolate and chocolate bars	−1	Plain chocolate	31
Corn chips	−1		20

224

Flavoured topping	−1	High in sugar	1
Fruit spreads	+1		0
Honey	+1		0
Jams and preserves	+1		0
Jellybeans	−1	High in sugar; converts to fat if unused	0
Liquorice	−1		2
Marshmallows	−1		0
Muesli bar	−1	Approx. 4–5 grams of fat in each bar	12
Nachos	−1		15
Pancakes	+1	Low in fat by themselves; high-fat toppings, e.g. ice cream, score −1	5
Peanut brittle	−1	High in fat	30
Peanut butter	−1	High in fat	50
Pretzels	+1	Unsalted	6
Popcorn	+1	Plain, microwaved	3
"	−1	Cooked in butter or oil	21
Potato chips	−1		34
Sesame crunch	−1		20
Syrup	−1	High in sugar; converts to fat if unused	0
Toffee	−1	Very high in sugar	5
Tortilla chips	−1		30
Twisties	−1		26

Biscuits and cookies

Arrowroot biscuits	0		4
Chocolate chip cookies	−1		10
Chocolate Tim Tams	−1		22

Chocolate wafers	−1		7
Crispbread	0		5
Custard cream	−1		18
Ginger nut biscuit	−1		7
Peanut crunch	−1		20
Plain sweet biscuits	−1		7
Shortbread	−1	High butter (fat) content	20
Sweet cream biscuits	−1		18
Wagon Wheel	−1		20

Cakes, pastries and puddings

Apple crumble	0		6
Apple pie	−1		15
Apple strudel	−1		20
Banana cake	−1		15
Black forest cake	−1		19
Bread and butter pudding	−1		18
Carrot cake	−1		20
Cheesecake	−1		23
Chocolate cake	−1	No cream	18
Chocolate éclair	−1	18 g of fat per éclair	18
Chocolate mud cake	−1		26
Chocolate pudding	−1		15
Christmas pudding	−1		10
Cream puff	−1		25
Creme caramel	−1		25
Custard tart	−1		15
Danish pastry	−1		15

Doughnut	−1	Iced	16
Fruit cake	−1		12
Fruit jelly	0	High in sugar	0
Gingerbread cake	−1		7
Icing	−1	e.g. chocolate/butter icing	6
Jam tarts	−1	1 jam tart weighs 50 g	15
Lamington	−1	Without cream, weighs 50 g	12
Lemon meringue pie	−1		10
Madeira cake	−1		15
Marble cake	−1		15
Mince pies	−1		16
Pastry	−1	Generally 20–30 g of fat; check packet before purchasing	
Filo	0	Low fat form of pastry	2
Pavlova	−1	With fruit and cream; high sugar content	8
Pecan pie	−1		22
Pineapple upside-down cake	−1		10
Rice pudding	−1		3
Scones	−1	With jam and cream	28
Sponge cake	−1	With cream	16
Tapioca pudding	−1		14
Trifle	−1		9
Vanilla slice	−1		10

Dressings and Sauces

Alfredo sauce	−1	Very high in fat	40
Barbecue sauce	0		0
Bolognese sauce	−1		12
"	0	Lean mince, no oil	6
Cream cheese sauce	−1	High in fat	35

Hollandaise sauce	−1		5
Italian sauces	+1	Bottled, e.g.: Leggo's, Dolmio's	<1
Mayonnaise	−1		32
Mornay sauce	−1		16
Mustard	0		2
Salad dressing French	−1		25
Salad dressing Italian	−1		32
Salad dressing Thousand Island	−1		22
Soy sauce	0	High in salt: minimal servings acceptable	0
Taco sauce	0		2
Tartar sauce	−1		27
Tomato sauce	0	High in salt and sugar: minimal servings acceptable	0
White sauce	−1		10

Margarines, oils and spreads

All vegetable oils are 100% fat.

Almond oil	−1		100
Canola oil	0		100
Grapeseed oil	0		100
Hazelnut oil	−1		100
Margarine/butter	−1		80
Olive oil	0	A type of monounsaturated fat; more desirable than polyunsaturated fats	100
Peanut oil	−1		100
Sesame oil	−1		100
Soya bean oil	−1		100
Sunflower oil	−1		100
Walnut oil	−1		100

Drinks

*The first two fruit juice drinks, alcohol, tea or coffee (including de caf.) and sports drinks score +1. Additional drinks score −1. Herbal teas count as +1 each time.

Apple juice	*		<1
Apricot nectar	*		<1
Cappuccino	*		3
Carrot juice	*		<1
Cocoa (hot chocolate)	−1		8
Coffee	*		3
Cranberry juice	*		<1
Fruit Smoothie	+1	Without ice cream or flavouring; must have fruit and yoghurt	2
Skim milk, Columbo	+1		0
Ginger ale	0		0
Grapefruit juice	*		3
Lemon juice	*		<1
Lime juice	*		<1
Malted milk	−1	Ice cream and milk create high fat content	8
Milkshake	−1	Standard	6
"	+1	Skim milk, yoghurt	1
Orange juice		*	<1
Passionfruit juice	*		<1
Peach nectar	*		7
Pineapple juice	*		2
Prune juice	*		<1
Soft drinks	−1	High in sugar	0
Sports drinks	*		<1
Tea (herbal)	+1		<1
Tea (with milk)	*		<1
Tomato juice	*		3
Tonic water	0		0

Water	+1	For first 8 glasses per day, then 0 for additional glasses	0
Water (mineral)	0	High in sugar	0
Whitener	−1	Non-dairy	34
Alcoholic beverages*		Alcohol has no fat content; alcoholic cocktails may include ingredients high in fat, e.g. Pina Colada	
Cigarettes	−1	For every cigarette smoked during the day	

Take-away food

Chinese

Beef and blackbean sauce	−1		8
Noodles	−1	Fried	12
Sweet and sour pork	−1		10
Vegetable stir fry	0		4
Prawn crackers	−1	Very high in fat	22

Greek

Falafel	+1		8
Kebabs	+1	1 kebab	6 per serve
Moussaka	−1		12

KFC

Burgers

Bacon and cheese (191 g)	−1		12 per serve
Chicken fillet (159 g)	−1		10 per serve
Colonel (114 g)	−1		14 per serve
Works burger (235 g)	−1		10 per serve
Zinger (179 g)	−1		9 per serve

Works Zinger (247 g)	−1		7 per serve
Chicken	−1		19
Chips	−1		20
Corn	+1		2
Desserts	−1		8
Potatoes and gravy	−1	Processed potatoes and butter	8
McDonald's			
Bacon and egg McMuffin	−1	Weighs approx. 140 g	20 per serve
Hashbrowns	−1	Weighs approx. 60 g	13 per serve
Hot cakes	−1	Weighs approx. 250 g	12 per serve
Burgers			
Big Mac (215 g)	−1		27 per serve
Quarter Pounder (200 g)	−1		36 per serve
Fillet O Fish (150 g)	−1		16 per serve
Cheese burger (115 g)	−1		16 per serve
Junior burger (100 g)	−1		11 per serve
Apple pie	−1		17 per serve
French fries	−1	Large serve (170 g)	26 per serve
McNuggets	−1	6 pack (115 g)	20 per seve
Red Rooster			
Chicken	−1		12
Chicken	+1	Skinless and grilled	3
Chips	−1		20
Desserts	−1		8
Ohter			
Chicko Roll	−1		10
Crab sticks	−1	Processed, preserved, high in fat	17
Dim sims (fried)	−1	One dim sim weighs 50 g	23

Food	Rating	Comments	Fat in grams
Dim sims (steamed)	−1	Highly processed, preserved	12
Fish and chips	−1		25
Hamburger	−1	Plain	10
"	−1	Egg, bacon, cheese	15
Pineapple/ Banana fritters	−1	Batter high in fat	20
Pizza	−1	Hawaiian	14
"	−1	Supreme	18
"	−1	The lot	21
Potato cakes	−1		15
Seafood stick	−1		17
Souvlaki	+1	Only if meat is lean, on a vertical griller	3
Spring rolls	−1		10
Steak sandwiches	−1	If oil, margarine, fatty meat used	20

FOOD LISTS (ALPHABETICAL ORDER)

Food	Rating	Comments	Fat in grams 100 (grams unless specified otherwise)
Alcoholic beverages	*	First 2 drinks = +1, −1 thereafter	0
Alfalfa sprouts	+1		0
Alfredo sauce	−1	Very high in fat	40
Almonds	−1		55
All Bran	+1		2
Almond oil	−1		100
Anchovies	−1	High in fat	14
Apple	+1		<1
Apple crumble	0		6
Apple juice	*		<1
Apple pie	−1		15
Apple strudel	−1		20
Apricot	+1		<1

Apricot nectar	*		<1
Arrowroot biscuits	0		4
Arrowroot flour	+1		0
Asparagus	+1		<1
Avocado	−1	High in fat	30
Bacon	−1		35
Bagel	+1	No butter	4 per bagel
Baked beans	+1		4
Bamboo shoots	+1		<1
Banana	+1		<1
Banana cake	−1		15
Banana fritter	−1		20
Barbecue sauce	0		0
Barbecued chicken	−1	With skin	13
"	+1	Skinless	8
Barley	+1		2
Barramundi	+1	Grilled, plain sauce	<1
Beans	+1		<1
Beef and blackbean sauce	−1		8
Beetroot	+1		<1
Black forest cake	−1		19
Black-eyed beans	+1		1
Blackberries	+1		<1
Blackcurrants	+1		<1
Boiled sweets	0		0
Bolognese sauce	−1		20
"	+1	No oil, lean meat	8
Brazil nuts	0		65
Bread and butter pudding	−1		18
Brie	−1		30

Broad beans	+1		<1
Broccoli	+1		<1
Brussel sprouts	+1		<1
Buckwheat flour	+1		2
Burger rings	−1		26
Butter	−1		82
Cabbage	+1		<1
Camembert	−1		28
Cannellini beans	+1		<1
Cannelloni	+1		1
Canola oil	0		100
Cappuccino	*		3
Carbonara	−1		12
Carob cookies	−1	High in fat	25
Carrot	+1		<1
Carrot cake	−1		20
Carrot juice	*		<1
Cashew nuts	−1	Salted	45
Cauliflower	+1		<1
Caviar	0		8
Celery	+1		<1
Cheddar	−1		38
Cheesecake	−1		23
Cheese and bacon balls	−1		34
Cheezles	−1		30
Cherries	+1		<1
Chestnuts	0		3
Chick peas	+1		2
Chicken Breast	−1	With skin	12
"	+1	Skinless, grilled	4
Chicken, fried	−1		17
Chicken parmigiana	−1	Made with ham and cheese	22

Food	Rating	Notes	Value
Chicko Roll	−1		10
Chicory	+1		<1
Chocolate and chocolate bars	−1	Plain chocolate	31
Chocolate cake	−1	No cream	18
Chocolate chip cookies	−1		10
Chocolate éclair	−1	18gms of fat per éclair	18
Chocolate mud cake	−1		26
Chocolate pudding	−1		15
Chocolate Tim Tams	−1		22
Chocolate wafers	−1		7
Christmas pudding	−1		10
Cigarettes	−1	For every cigarette smoked during the day	
Cocoa (hot chocolate)	−1		8
Coco Pops	0	Contain more sugar than most cereals	<1
Coconut	−1	Fresh	27
"	−1	Dessicated	62
Cod	+1	Grilled, plain sauce	<1
Coffee	*		3
Columbo ice cream	+1	A low fat variety of ice cream	8
Corn chips	−1		20
Cornflakes	+1		1
Cornflour	+1		<1
Cottage cheese	+1	Low in fat	14
Crab	+1		1
Crab sticks	−1	Processed, preserved, high in fat	17
Cranberry juice	*		<1
Crayfish	+1		1

Cream	−1		35
Cream cheese sauce	−1	High in fat	35
Cream puffs	−1		25
Creme caramel	−1		25
Crispbread	0		5
Croissant	−1	Pastry high in fat	16
Crumpets	+1		2 per serve
Crunchy nut corn flakes	0		4
Cucumber	+1		<1
Currants	+1		<1
Custard cream	−1		18
Danish pastry	−1		15
Dark rye bread	+1		1 per slice
Dates	+1		<1
Dim sims (fried)	−1	1 dim sim weighs 50 g	23
Dim sims (steamed)	−1	Highly processed, preserved	12
Doner kebab	+1	Low fat take-away option	6
Doughnut	−1	Iced	16
Duck	0	Roast, skinless	10
"	−1	Roast, with skin	29
Eggplant	+1		2
Eggs	*	First two for the week count as +1	11
Fried	−1		18
Scrambled	−1		14
Falafel	+1		8
Fennel	+1		<1
Feta cheese	−1		30
Fettucini	+1		<1

Food	Rating	Comment	Fat
Figs	+1		<1
Filo pastry	0	Low fat form of pastry	2
Fish and chips	−1	Very high in fat	25
Fish fingers	−1	Pre-fried, high in preservatives	16
Flake	+1	Grilled, plain sauce	1
Flathead	+1	Grilled, plain sauce	1
Flavoured topping	−1	High in sugar	1
Flounder	+1	Grilled, plain sauce	<1
Focaccia	−1		7
Frankfurters	−1		13
Fruit cake	−1		12
Fruit jelly	0	High in sugar	0
Fruit salad	+1		<1
Fruit smoothie	+1	Without ice cream or flavouring; must have fruit and yoghurt	2
Fruit spreads	+1		0
Garlic	+1		<1
Garlic bread	−1	Use of butter, high fat content	18
Garlic prawns	−1		9
Gherkins	+1		<1
Ginger	+1		<1
Ginger ale	0		0
Ginger nut biscuit	−1		7
Gingerbread cake	−1		7
Gnocchi	+1	Potato gnocchi with cheese	1
Grapefruit	+1		<1
Grapefruit juice	*		3
Grapes	+1		<1
Grapeseed oil	0		100
Green beans	+1		<1
Guava	+1		<1

Haddock	+1	Grilled, plain sauce	1
Ham	0	Can be high in fat	5
Hamburgers	−1	Plain	10
"	−1	Egg, bacon, cheese	15
Haricot beans	+1		1
Hazelnut oil	−1		100
Hazelnuts	−1		61
Heart	0	Not fried	16
Herring	−1	High in fat	14
Hollandaise sauce	−1		5
Honey	+1		0
Hot dog	−1	High in fat, preservatives	15
Ice cream	−1		24
Icing	−1	e.g. chocolate/butter icing	6
Italian sauces	+1	Bottled, e.g. Leggo's, Dolmio's	<1
Jam tarts	−1	One jam tart weighs 50 g	15
Jams and preserves	+1		0
Jellybeans	−1	High in sugar	0
Just Right	+1		1
Kidney	0	Not fried.	16
Kidney beans	+1		<1
Kiwi fruit	+1		<1
KFC			
Bacon and cheese burger (191 g)	−1		12 per serve
Chicken fillet burger (159 g)	−1		10 per serve
Colonel burger (114 g)	−1		14 per serve

Works burger (235 g)	−1		10 per serve
Zinger burger (179 g)	−1		9 per serve
Works zinger burger (247 g)	−1		7 per serve
Chicken	−1		19
Chips	−1		20
Corn	+1		2
Desserts	−1		8
Potatoes and gravy	−1	Processed potatoes and butter	8
Lamb chops	−1		31
"	0	Grilled, lean	12
Lamington	−1	Without cream, weight 50 g	12
Lasagna	0	With meat	6
"	+1	With vegetables	4
Leeks	+1		<1
Lemon juice	*		<1
Lemon meringue pie	−1		10
Lemons	+1		<1
Lentils	+1		<1
Lettuce	+1		<1
Light rye	+1		1 per slice
Lima beans	+1		<1
Lime juice	*		<1
Liquorice	−1		2
Liver	0	Not fried	16
Lobster	+1		1
Lychees	+1		<1
Macadamia nuts	−1		76
Macaroni	−1	Baked with cheese	13
"	+1	Wholewheat, no cheese	2

Mackerel	0		10
Madeira cake	−1		15
Malted milk	−1		8
Mandarins	+1		<1
Mangoes	+1		<1
Marble cake	−1		15
Margarine	−1		80
Marshmallows	−1		0
Mayonnaise	−1		32
McDonald's			
Bacon and egg McMuffin	−1	Weighs approx. 140 g	20 per serve
Hashbrowns	−1	Weighs approx. 60 g	13 per serve
Hot cakes	−1	Weighs approx. 250 g	12 per serve
Burgers	−1	Big Mac (215 g)	27 per serve
Quarter Pounder (200 g)	−1		36 per serve
Fillet O Fish (150 g)	−1		16 per serve
Cheese burger (115 g)	−1		16 per serve
Junior burger (100 g)	−1		11 per serve
Apple pie	−1	17 per serve	
French fries	−1	Large serve (170 g)	26 per serve
McNuggets	−1	6 pack (115 g)	20 per serve
Meat pie	−1	At least 20 g of fat per pie	20+
Melon	+1		<1
Milk			
Skim	+1		0
Physical/Rev	0		20
Whole	−1		40
Soy	0	Still relatively high in fat	16
Milkshake	−1	Standard	6
"	+1	Skim milk, yoghurt	1

Mince beef	−1		10
"	+1	Extra lean	6
Mince pies	−1		16
Mornay sauce	−1		16
Moussaka	−1		12
Mozzarella cheese	−1		30
Muesli	−1	Toasted, high in fat	25
"	+1	Natural	5
Muesli bar	−1	Approx. 4–5 g fat in each bar	12
Muffins	+1	Per small muffin	3
Multi-grain bread	+1		1 per slice
Mung beans	+1		<1
Mushrooms	+1		<1
Mussels	0		2
Mustard	0		2
Naan	−1		7 per serve
Nachos	−1		15
Nectarines	+1		<1
Noodles	−1	Fried	12
Oat bran	+1		3
Oat meal	+1		7
Octopus (calamari)	+1	If fried score −1	1
Olive oil	0		100
Olives	+1		2
Onions	+1		<1
Orange juice	*		<1
Oranges	+1		<1
Oyster	0		1
Pancakes	+1		5
Parmesan cheese	−1		28

Parsnip	+1		<1
Passionfruit	+1		<1
Passionfruit juice	*		<1
Pastry	−1		20–30
Pavlova	−1	With fruit and cream	8
Paw-paw	+1		<1
Peach nectar	*		7
Peaches	+1		<1
Peanuts	−1	Roasted, unsalted	49
"	−1	Roasted, salted	49
Peanut brittle	−1	High in fat	30
Peanut butter	−1	High in fat	50
Peanut crunch	−1		20
Peanut oil	−1		100
Pears	+1		<1
Peas	+1		<1
Pecan nuts	−1		71
Pecan pie	−1		22
Peppers	+1		<1
Pilchards	+1	Steamed	3
Pineapple	+1		<1
Pineapple fritter	−1	Batter high in fat	20
Pineapple juice	*		2
Pineapple upside-down cake	−1		10
Pine nuts	−1		51
Pinto beans	+1		2
Pistachio nuts	−1	Shelled	48
"	−1	Unshelled	28
Pitta bread	+1		2
Pizza	−1	Hawaiian	14
"	−1	Supreme	18
"	−1	The lot	21

Plums	+1		<1
Popcorn	+1	Plain, microwaved	3
"	−1	Cooked in butter or oil	21
Pork, new fashioned	+1		9
Porridge	+1		5
Porterhouse steak	−1	Tends to have high fat content	15
"	+1	Small, grilled, lean, trimmed	8
Potato cakes	−1		15
Potato chips	−1		34
Potatoes	+1		<1
"	+1	Dry baked in jackets	0
"	−1	Fried in oil; thick cut (>1cm thick)	14
"	−1	Roasted in oil	5
"	0	Mashed with butter or margerine	8
Prawn crackers	−1	Very high in fat	22
Prawns	+1		2
Pretzels	+1	Unsalted	6
Prune juice	*		<1
Prunes	+1		<1
Pumpkin	+1		<1
"	−1	Roasted in oil	6
Radish	+1		<1
Raisin bread	+1		1 per slice
Raisins	+1		<1
Raspberries	+1		<1
Ravioli	0	Meat filled	5
"	+1	Spinach and ricotta	3
Red Rooster			
Chicken	−1		12
Chicken	+1	Skinless and grilled	3
Chips	−1		20
Desserts	−1		8

Rhubarb	+1		<1
Rice	+1	Brown, boiled or steamed	1
"	−1	Brown, fried	7
"	+1	White, boiled or steamed	<1
"	−1	White, fried	6
Rice bubbles	+1		<1
Rice pudding	−1		3
Ricecakes	+1		<1
Ricotta	+1	Low in fat	12
Risotto	+1		4
Rump steak	−1	Tends to have high fat content	15
"	+1	Small, grilled, lean, trimmed	5
Rye flour	+1		3
Salad dressing (French)	−1		25
Salad dressing (Italian)	−1		32
Salad dressing (Thousand Island)	−1		22
Salami	−1	High in fat	45
Salmon	+1	No oil	5
Sardine	−1	Canned in oil, not drained	28
"	−1	Cannned in oil, drained	14
Sausage roll	−1		18
Sausages	−1		13
Scallops	+1		1
Scones	−1	With jam and cream	28
Seafood stick	−1		17
Semolina	+1		1
Sesame crunch	−1		20
Sesame oil	−1		100
Sesame seeds	−1		50
Shortbread	−1		20

Silverside	−1		15
Sirloin steak	−1		12
"	+1	Lean, trimmed and grilled	8
Snapper	+1	Grilled, plain sauce	1
Soft drinks	−1	High in sugar	0
Sour cream	−1		18
Sourdough bread	+1		1 per slice
Souvlaki	+1	Only if meat is lean, on vertical griller	3
Soya beans	+1		6
Soy and linseed bread	+1		3 per slice
Soybean flour	−1	Full fat	17
"	+1	Low fat	1
Soya bean oil	−1		100
Soy sauce	0	High in salt	0
Spaghetti	+1	Plain	<1
"	+1	Wholewheat	<1
Spaghetti bolognese	−1	With oil	15
Special K	+1		1
Spinach	+1		<1
Sponge cake	−1	With cream	16
Sports drinks	*		<1
Spring onions	+1		<1
Spring rolls	−1		10
Steak sandwiches	−1	If oil, margarine, fatty meat used	20
Stir fry vegetables	0		4
Strassburg	−1		24
Strawberries	+1		<1
Sultana Bran	+1		1
Sultanas	+1		<1
Sunflower oil	−1		100
Sunflower seeds	−1		50
Sustain	+1		3

Sweet and sour pork	−1		10
Sweet biscuits (plain)	−1		7
Sweet cream biscuits	−1		18
Sweetcorn	+1		<1
Swiss cheese	−1		30
Syrup	−1		0
Taco sauce	0		2
Taco shells	0		4 per shell
Tangerines	+1		<1
Tapioca pudding	−1		14
Tartar sauce	−1		27
T-bone steak	−1	Tend to have high fat content	12
Tea (herbal)	+1		<1
Tea (with milk)	*		<1
Toffee	−1	Also very high in sugar	5
Tofu	0		8
"	−1	Fried	16
Tomato juice	*		3
Tomato sauce	0	High in salt and sugar	0
Tomatoes	+1		<1
Tonic water	0		0
Tortellini	0		8
Tortilla chips	−1		30
Trifle	−1		9
Trout	+1	Grilled, plain sauce	3
Tuna	+1	Brine, water	3
"	−1	Canned in oil	22
Turkey	+1		3
Twisties	−1		26

Food		Note	Value
Vanilla slice	−1		10
Veal	+1	Lean, grilled	4
Veal parmigiana	−1		20
Vitari	0		10
Walnut oil	−1		100
Wagon Wheel	−1		20
Walnuts	0	Helps protect against heart disease	52
Water	+1	For each of 8 glasses per day	0
Water (mineral)	0	High in sugar	0
Water biscuits	0	Fat content varies, read label	
Weetbix	+1		2
Wheatgerm	+1		6
White bread	+1		1 per slice
White fibre-increased bread	+1		2 per slice
White sauce	−1		10
Whitener	−1	Non-dairy	34
Whiting	+1	Grilled, plain sauce	1
Wholemeal bread	+1		2 per slice
Wholewheat flour	+1		2
Wild rice	+1		3
Yoghurt	+1	Low fat	6
"	0	Regular	16
Zucchini	+1		<1

Appendix 3:
Every Day Counts diary

'A verbal contract isn't worth the paper it's written on.'

WHY USE THE DIARY?

Recording your scores on a daily basis is essential. You have to establish a routine and recording your scores is a vital part of that routine. It's too easy to change your mind when nothing's committed to paper. This Appendix provides pages to be reproduced so that you can monitor your progress.

Your Every Day Counts experience is designed to last for 9 months. After 9 months of living in the Health Zone you will no longer need a system because positive health practices will be an integral part of your daily lifestyle. You will be eating a low-fat diet, exercising regularly and managing stress as a matter of habit.

Along the way you will require some discipline to keep you on track and up to date. Recording your daily points scores will ensure that your actions are matching your commitments. It's a simple yet vital way to keep yourself on schedule. Recording your daily achievements puts a deadline on your goal of a healthy and vibrant lifestyle. When you write something down it automatically becomes more significant than when it exists only as a thought.

Writing down your daily scores is a proven means of keeping yourself 'with the program'. It's vital that you not only follow the system, but that you record yourself following the system.

HOW TO USE THE DIARY

There are four sections to the diary.

The first enables you to get used to the system during your 2-week trial. There are no targets or requirements during this trial; it's simply an opportunity to experiment with recording your daily points scores.

The second section is dedicated to the vital first 7 days after you commence the program. Here you record daily food, exercise and pressure points for the first time in earnest.

The third section provides space to record your daily scores during the 7 consecutive weeks of Every Day Counts.

The fourth and final section will provide you with a record of your points scores each day for the 7 months that then follow.

In summary, the diary sections are:

	Days	Weeks	Months
Section 1:	14 day trial	2	-
Section 2:	1 to 7	1	-
Section 3:	8 to 56	2 to 8	1 to 2
Section 4:	57 to 253*	9 to 36	3 to 9

*In Every Day Counts, a month is exactly 4 weeks. Every 28 days sees the beginning of a new month.

FILLING IN YOUR DIARY

1   REWARDS

Before you start the program, decide what your daily, weekly and monthly rewards are going to be. Please record these in the spaces provided for the complete duration of the program, before you start Day One.

Here are 7 ideas for daily, weekly and monthly rewards:

Daily rewards: Breakfast in bed, favourite meal, hiring a video, sex, sleeping in, buying a magazine, raffle or lottery ticket.

Weekly rewards: Pay for a professional massage, see a new release movie or show, go out for a meal, buy a book that you've wanted, have a food or drink treat, have some chores done for you (lawn mowing, ironing, window cleaning), buy yourself a favourite CD or tape.

Monthly rewards: Have your car detailed inside and out, buy yourself a piece of jewellery, an item of clothing or a pair of new shoes. Have a night or weekend away by yourself, with your partner or a friend. As your final monthly reward purchase a trinket that will remind you of what you have achieved. This should be something you look at rather than something you use for a specific function. It is a symbol of what you will have achieved.

These are only ideas, so go ahead and design your own reward package. There is no set guide to how much you should spend. Your daily rewards might have a value of 1 dollar or a value of up to 10 dollars each. It's completely up to you and your own circumstances. Whatever you spend will be a great investment in yourself.

2   DAILY RECORDS

There are spaces provided for you to record your food points, exercise points and pressure points in each section of the diary. You will find pages for you to reproduce for each of the 4 sections of the program. You may wish to create your own complete diary before you start the program. This will enable you to record your rewards up to the final month.

Rather than have to carry a pen and paper around with you each day, the simplest method is to think back and score yourself at the end of each day. You will inevitably find that you will keep progressive scores in your mind. This tends to happen automatically, almost subconsciously. When it comes time for your after-dinner snack, you will find yourself thinking something like this: 'Well, I've had 23 food choices, I'm sitting on 11 points and I've had approximately 48 grams of fat. I had better make my snack a piece of fruit because I need a positive point and I don't have any grams of fat to spare.'

Other nights you will find yourself thinking, 'I'm up to 24 food choices, I'm already on 13 points and I've only had 30 grams of fat. I can afford a negative point and I have some grams to spare. Where's the chocolate?' These are the nights you will find that chocolate has never tasted better or more satisfying!

At day's end, just think back and fill in the 3 figures you need. This is your food score, your exercise score and your pressure score. Add the 3 scores together and write in your total. On exercise days, your total points target is 20 and on non-exercise days your points target is 16. That's all it takes to fill in your daily record, a maximum of 3 minutes, probably less, each day. The first habit you need to develop is the habit of filling in your daily record each night.

A lot of people keep their diary in a drawer in their bathroom so that it is always in the same place. At night when they are about to clean their teeth before going to bed, they fill in their points score for the day. This makes it easy to remember, part of a nightly routine. Please make it part of your nightly ritual.

3 HUMANITY DAYS
You may recall that you have 1 'humanity day' each week. This means that as long as you reach your points target on 6 out of every 7 days, you will be succeeding!

You can record your humanity days by simply writing in an 'H' on any day you allocate as a humanity day. Still record your points score for that day, even if it ends up being a lonely, small single figure (like 1 point). The more you record what you achieve, the more valuable the experience will be for you. Remember that it's 1 humanity day per week, no more. Don't be reluctant to use them. They have been designed into the program for a specific purpose and you will find times when you do need them. Use them.

A final word on humanity days. They are not cumulative. You cannot save them up or hold them over from weeks when you don't use them. Don't take them just because they are there unless you are feeling the need for a let-down. Humanity days are a reserve and an escape clause. Use them wisely.

POINTS DIARY

SECTION ONE: 14-DAY TRIAL

WEEK ONE

	FOOD	EXERCISE	PRESSURE	TOTAL
Monday				
Tuesday				
Wednesday				
Thursday				
Friday				
Saturday				
Sunday				

WEEK TWO

	FOOD	EXERCISE	PRESSURE	TOTAL
Monday				
Tuesday				
Wednesday				
Thursday				
Friday				
Saturday				
Sunday				

POINTS DIARY

SECTION TWO: DAYS 1–7

WEEK ONE

	FOOD	EXERCISE	PRESSURE	TOTAL
Monday				

Reward: _____

	FOOD	EXERCISE	PRESSURE	TOTAL
Tuesday				

Reward: _____

	FOOD	EXERCISE	PRESSURE	TOTAL
Wednesday				

Reward: _____

	FOOD	EXERCISE	PRESSURE	TOTAL
Thursday				

Reward: _____

	FOOD	EXERCISE	PRESSURE	TOTAL
Friday				

Reward: _____

	FOOD	EXERCISE	PRESSURE	TOTAL
Saturday				

Reward: _____

	FOOD	EXERCISE	PRESSURE	TOTAL
Sunday				

Reward: _____

Humanity Day: _____

Total Weekly Points Target = 128 (4 days x 20 & 3 days x 16)

Actual =

POINTS DIARY

SECTION THREE: WEEKS 2–8

Reproduce the following pages as needed to create your diary for this section.

WEEK _ _ _

	FOOD	EXERCISE	PRESSURE	TOTAL
Monday				
Tuesday				
Wednesday				
Thursday				
Friday				
Saturday				
Sunday				
Total Weekly Points Target: 128			Your Total:	

Humanity Day: _____

Reward (Week ___): _____

WEEK _ _ _

	FOOD	EXERCISE	PRESSURE	TOTAL
Monday				
Tuesday				
Wednesday				
Thursday				
Friday				
Saturday				
Sunday				
Total Weekly Points Target: 128		Your Total:		

Humanity Day: _____

Reward (Week _ _ _): _____

POINTS DIARY

SECTION FOUR: MONTHS 3–9, WEEKS 9–36

Each month consists of 28 days. Reproduce these pages as needed to form your diary.

Rewards

Record your monthly rewards below, before you start your program.

Third month _____

Fourth month _____

Fifth month _____

Sixth month _____

Seventh month _____

Eighth month _____

Final reward _____

WEEK _ _ _

	FOOD	EXERCISE	PRESSURE	TOTAL
Monday				
Tuesday				
Wednesday				
Thursday				
Friday				
Saturday				
Sunday				
Total Weekly Points Target: 128		Your Total:		

Humanity Day: _____

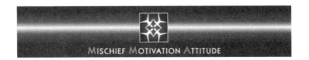

MISCHIEF MOTIVATION ATTITUDE

Mark McKeon's company, Mischief, Motivation, Attitude conducts Conference, Coaching and ongoing Training Programs in Wellbeing, Leadership and High Performing Teams. For more information please contact Derek Percival, Scott Mackay or Shane Garner at info@mckeon.com.au or go to www.mckeon.com.au

Mark is also the author of 'Work a Little Less, Live a Little More' and 'Mark McKeon's Life Tips'. Mark's books have been translated into Chinese and Portuguese and are widely published from Asia to South America. Copies of Mark's books are available from www.markmckeon.com

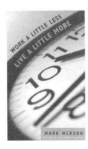
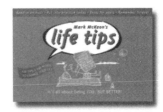

Mark's philosophy is that we should take no pride in doing something well if we shouldn't be doing it at all. Mark lives with his wife Carole and sons Jake and Sam, sharing time between their homes in Eltham and Ocean Grove in Victoria, Australia.

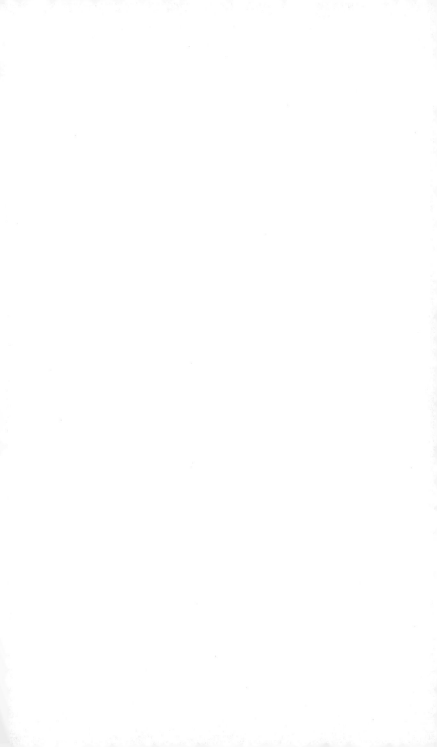

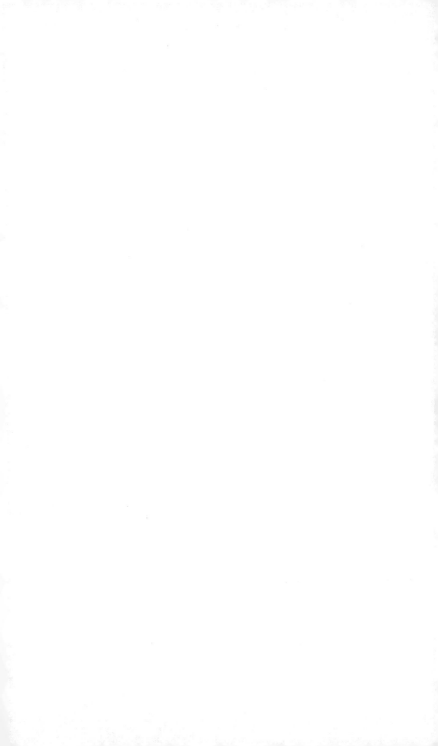

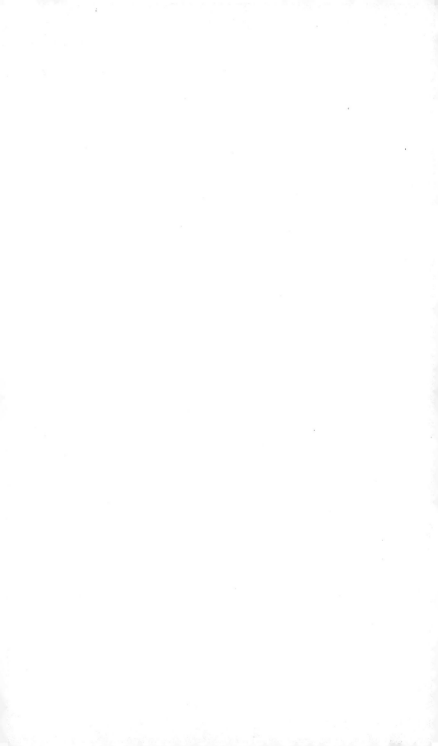